EASING THE PAIN
OF ARTHRITIS
Naturally

Everything You Need to Know to
Combat Arthritis Safely and Effectively

EARL L. MINDELL, R.PH., PH.D.

T0273477

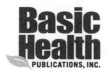

Basic
Health
PUBLICATIONS, INC.

The information contained in this book is based upon the research and personal and professional experiences of the author. It is not intended as a substitute for consulting with your physician or other healthcare provider. Any attempt to diagnose and treat an illness should be done under the direction of a healthcare professional.

The publisher does not advocate the use of any particular healthcare protocol but believes the information in this book should be available to the public. The publisher and author are not responsible for any adverse effects or consequences resulting from the use of the suggestions, preparations, or procedures discussed in this book. Should the reader have any questions concerning the appropriateness of any procedures or preparation mentioned, the author and the publisher strongly suggest consulting a professional healthcare advisor.

Basic Health Publications, Inc.
28812 Top of the World Drive
Laguna Beach, CA 92651
949-715-7327

Library of Congress Cataloging-in-Publication Data

Mindell, Earl.
   Easing the pain of arthritis naturally : everything you need to know to combat arthritis safely and effectively / Earl L. Mindell.
      p. cm.
   Includes bibliographical references and index.
   ISBN 1-59120-109-8 (alk. paper)
   1. Arthritis–Popular works. I. Title.

   RC933.M5655   2005
   616.7'22–dc22

                                        2004026323

Editor: Carol Rosenberg
Typesetting/Book design: Gary A. Rosenberg
Cover design: Mike Stromberg

Printed in the United States of America

10   9   8   7   6   5   4   3   2   1

Contents

Introduction

rthritis has reached epidemic proportions in developed nations. Approximately 80 million people worldwide suffer from chronic pain and inflammation in their joints, and this number continues to increase. In their search for relief, arthritis sufferers typically use over-the-counter and prescription medications. Some may visit physical therapists for costly treatments that only temporarily relieve discomfort. Others with severe cases may opt to undergo surgery, while still others simply choose to bear the pain.

Modern medicine has not yet found a cure for arthritis, and through the process of trying to find one, it has created an entirely new set of problems. Each year, an estimated 100,000 people are hospitalized and 16,000 patients die from side effects caused by commonly prescribed arthritis medications. The need for safer treatment methods has inspired an ongoing flurry of research and drug development by pharmaceutical companies. Recently, new arthritis medications that are touted as having minimal side effects are becoming available through the Federal Drug Administration's (FDA's) "fast-track" approval process. It remains to be seen, however, if these "miracles of science" have long-term effectiveness.

In this book, you'll learn everything you need to know about arthritis and how to combat it safely and effectively. Chapter 1 provides basic information on arthritis—what it is, how it develops, and the lifestyle changes that can help keep its painful symptoms to a minimum. As it is important to understand the actual causes of inflammation, Chapter 2 presents the process that causes joints to ache and swell. Nonsteroidal

1

anti-inflammatory drugs and COX-2 inhibitors—the drugs prescribed for alleviating arthritis pain—are discussed in Chapter 3. The drawbacks of these and other common drugs prescribed for arthritis also are discussed here. Subsequent chapters focus on many nutritional and complementary treatments that can ease arthritis pain and inflammation, including supplements, herbs (particularly ginger), alternative therapies, and exercise. In these chapters, you'll learn about safe, effective natural remedies that work synergistically with your body's natural tendency toward healing and balance, rather than against them.

The right natural remedies for arthritis—along with other steps to bring your body to a state of good health—can keep you off prescription drugs and out of the hospital. You'll soon learn that it *is* within your power to ease the pain of arthritis naturally.

CHAPTER 1

What Is Arthritis?

*T*he word *arthritis* means "inflammation of the joints." Arthritis strikes connective tissues in the body, causing joint pain, swelling, degeneration, and disability. There are more than one hundred types of arthritic disease, some of which affect only the joints and others that have more widespread effects. The two major types of arthritic disease are *osteoarthritis,* also known as *degenerative* arthritis; and *rheumatoid* arthritis, also known as *autoimmune* or *inflammatory* arthritis. Almost all of the arthritic diseases fall into one of these two categories. The onset, progression, and symptoms of rheumatoid arthritis and osteoarthritis are quite different, and they usually affect people in different age groups.

In this chapter, you'll learn about how your joints work and how arthritis can affect them. Understanding your joints, and what can go wrong with these marvels of engineering, is a prerequisite to knowing how best to support their health. Once you've learned the basics, you'll be able to grasp the rest of the information in this book much more easily, and you'll also be able to talk more easily with your healthcare practitioner about managing your arthritis.

HOW JOINTS WORK

Arthritis is a disease of the *connective tissues.* The entire human body is held together by connective tissues: Fasciae hold the muscles and organs in place and in their proper shapes; ligaments attach bones to one another; fat cushions and supports the organs and bones; and tendons

3

(dense, strong strips of connective tissue) connect the muscle to the bone. Other connective tissues, called cartilage, synovial membranes, and bursae also provide cushioning and lubrication between the ends of bones.

Connective tissue is made from tightly wound strands of protein called *collagen.* Specialized cells called *chondroblasts* secrete a matrix of carbohydrate and protein molecules into the grid formed by collagen fibers, providing a framework for other proteins, minerals, and fluids to fill in. When collagen fiber grids are filled in with minerals, it creates bones; when they are filled in with varying amounts of other proteins and fluids, cartilage, tendons, ligaments, fascia, and membranes are the result.

Cartilage is a layer of dense connective tissue that cushions joints, decreasing friction between bones. Smooth, firm, and flexible, cartilage can withstand a great deal of pressure, and springs right back to its original shape when the pressure is removed. Cartilage is a living, growing tissue. It contains no blood vessels but is nourished by the fluids that bathe the joints. These fluids move through the cartilage when the joint is moved. Without this regular nutrient bath, cartilage deteriorates.

Two types of joints can be affected by arthritis—synovial and cartilaginous. Both types contain a considerable amount of cartilage, which deteriorates in arthritis. *Synovial joints* include the major joints of the arms and legs. The inner surface of this type of joint is lined with a membrane that produces *hyaluronic acid,* a synovial fluid that lubricates the joint surfaces—much in the same way motor oil lubricates an engine—and allows the head of the bone to move freely in the socket. Some joints, such as the knee and the jaw, include cartilage discs that divide the synovial fluid into two compartments and that cushion the movement of the joint. The synovial fluid carries nutrients into the cartilage and keeps the cartilage surfaces of the joint separate from one another. *Cartilaginous joints* include the joints between the vertebrae. Between most of the vertebrae of the spine, round cushions of cartilage—often called *discs*—prevent the contact of bone with bone and give the spine its amazing range of movement.

OSTEOARTHRITIS

Osteoarthritis, the most common form of arthritis, affects an estimated 10 percent of the population worldwide. Almost 80 percent of people over age fifty have some degree of osteoarthritis. Believed to be caused primarily by wear and tear, osteoarthritis typically affects weight-bearing joints, such as those of the hips, knees, and spine. And because the hands are in constant use, the finger joints are often affected as well.

Osteoarthritis rarely involves the process of *inflammation,* and so the name "arthritis" isn't exactly appropriate for this joint disease. As the joint deteriorates, the synovial membrane becomes irritated and over-produces synovial fluid, causing swelling in the joint spaces. Sometimes this swelling is referred to as inflammation, although it rarely involves common symptoms of inflammation such as visible changes in the joint, heat, or involvement of the immune system. The irritation caused by friction between joint surfaces simply causes the synovial membrane to make more fluid than the joint can hold.

Generally, osteoarthritis is considered a disease of aging. In it, the spongy, flexible cartilage that cushions areas where bone meets bone begins to wear. In aging cartilage, protein-digesting enzymes dramatically increase their rate of activity, leading to rapid deterioration of cartilage. The body can't replace it fast enough, especially an aging body that does-n't make cartilage as well as it used to. As a result, the surfaces within the joint no longer slide over one another smoothly. Once like the perfectly matched pieces of a jigsaw puzzle, the roughened joint surfaces begin to rasp against one another. (Imagine trying to screw an improperly aligned lid on a jar—when you turn it, the lid and the jar grind against each other rather than the surfaces gliding smoothly over one another.) In cases of advanced osteoarthritis, the body summons its healing forces to try to repair the joint, and inflammation, along with the resulting pain, swelling, redness, and heat, can occur.

At first, osteoarthritis pain strikes only when the affected joint is being used, but after a while, the joint starts to hurt constantly. As the cartilage wears away, the body tries to repair the joint by building new bone and cartilage. If, however, these structures are not aligned properly, painful bone spurs that reduce range of motion may result.

Men are much more likely than women to develop osteoarthritis young, but women are ten times more likely to develop it than men after the age of forty-five. Nearly every person over the age of sixty-five shows some evidence of cartilage deterioration, especially in the weight-bearing joints of the hips, spine, and knees. Only about one-third of them ever have arthritis symptoms, however. This is a good indication that there are factors in play in osteoarthritis that have little to do with the amount of cartilage in the joints. Although we don't know exactly what those factors are, they may explain why certain natural remedies work to relieve the symptoms of the disease.

There are actually several types of osteoarthritis. The most common forms include:

- *Bursitis.* Painful swelling of the *bursae*—small sacs found in the connective tissue, usually near joints. These sacs are filled with synovial fluid, which reduces friction between tendons and bones or ligaments. Often, bursitis is the result of prolonged stress or pressure that causes the bursae to become inflamed or swollen. Once inflamed, the swollen sacs press against a neighboring joint, creating pain.

- *Tendonitis.* Painful swelling of a *tendon*—fibrous tissue that attaches muscle to bone. Usually this inflammation is caused by overexertion in sports or other physical activity. Tendonitis commonly occurs in the tendons found in the knee, elbow, and rotator cuff, which stabilizes the shoulder. The Achilles tendon, located at the back of the ankle, also is commonly affected.

- *Carpal tunnel syndrome.* A condition resulting from excessive or repetitive pressure on the median nerve, located in the hand. The median nerve, which controls some of the hand and finger muscles, passes through a tiny opening located below the wrist called the carpal tunnel. Repetitious movement involving the wrist and fingers creates irritation and swelling, which causes the tissue of the carpal tunnel to press on the median nerve. Tingling, numbness, and pain are common symptoms. The repetitive finger motion caused by constantly typing or punching keys on a computer keyboard can cause carpal tunnel syndrome.

- *Fibromyalgia.* A disorder that is characterized by muscle and joint pain without any inflammation that persists for no apparent reason. The cause of this condition, which affects about 10 million Americans and is closely associated with chronic fatigue syndrome, is not clearly understood.

In osteoarthritis, there appears to be a genetic factor at play. Those who develop osteoarthritis in their forties or sooner are likely to have other family members who also did. This could have to do with family members having similar joint structures that are more vulnerable to wear and tear. Those with such a predisposition should take preventive measures against osteoarthritis, including regular strengthening and stretching exercises, proper diet, and attention to good posture—preferably under the guidance of a physical therapist.

Others who may be prone to osteoarthritis are those whose occupations demand sitting in chairs or vehicles for much of the day. Years of this type of posture, coupled with lack of proper exercise, commonly causes the hips and spine to become misaligned. In turn, the joints in the legs and neck also are knocked out of proper alignment, resulting in stress on the cartilaginous surfaces within the joints.

Repetitive stress on certain joints also increases the risk of osteoarthritis. Athletes, dancers, and those who do repetitive physical labor are at risk of wearing away the cartilage in the joints they use most. But don't think that lying around like a couch potato will protect you from osteoarthritis, either. Those who don't get proper exercise are at increased risk as well. Joints that are not moved regularly through their full range of motion are far more likely to deteriorate with age.

Other known risk factors for osteoarthritis include obesity and smoking. Poor postural habits can also throw joints out of alignment and cause uneven stresses on cartilage and other connective tissues. And if you have injured a joint, there is a greater likelihood of that area becoming arthritic.

There is no cure for osteoarthritis. Although cartilage can rebuild itself, there is no surefire way to reverse the process that destroyed the joint in the first place. Living with chronic pain can be a waking nightmare. Especially painful is arthritis that affects the intervertebral discs of the spine. Muscles tighten and nerves can become entrapped. If you have ever suffered from back pain, you know that when your back hurts, it's hard to function. Each year, back pain is responsible for putting 7 million people temporarily out of work.

Most approaches for arthritis involve controlling the pain and inflammation with drugs and allowing the body to heal itself to the best of its ability. The most common drugs for alleviating the painful symptoms of osteoarthritis include nonsteroidal anti-inflammatory drugs (NSAIDs) and steroid drugs like cortisone. In Chapter 3, you'll learn more about these drugs and their harmful side effects, and you will also see why natural remedies are superior alternatives.

Arthroscopic surgery is a treatment method for relieving friction within arthritic joints. Through this procedure, a tiny catheter is introduced into the joint where it smoothes out bumpy cartilage surfaces. In very severe cases, arthritic joints are surgically replaced with artificial ones. Although these procedures have helped many people deal with arthritis, any surgical procedure has inherent risks. In many cases, they need to be repeated. Surgery also is expensive and, in arthritis cases, should be considered only by those who are crippled by the disease. (Chapter 3 has more on common surgical procedures for arthritis.)

RHEUMATOID ARTHRITIS

Rheumatoid arthritis (RA), also referred to as inflammatory arthritis, strikes about 3 million Americans. It is three to five times more common in women than men, and primarily affects young people between ages twenty and fifty. Infants and children can also suffer from rheumatoid arthritis. It is most common in Westernized countries and all but unknown in less developed nations. Some people with rheumatoid arthritis recover from their first bout and never have it again. Others have long periods of remission between flare-ups, and some struggle against the disease more or less constantly.

Rheumatoid arthritis is categorized as an autoimmune disorder. In it, the immune system mistakenly attacks the body's own tissues, causing chronic and damaging levels of inflammation, pain, and joint swelling. Joints of the hands, feet, wrists, knees, hips, and ankles most commonly are affected. Initially, a joint's synovial membranes become inflamed, which cause it to swell and become stiff. As a result, the inflamed membranes emit enzymes that break down joint cartilage. The cartilage is replaced by fibrous tissue, which can calcify and form bony knobs that may fuse the joint, restricting movement.

Within the joint spaces affected by rheumatoid arthritis, immune cells called *lymphocytes* react to what they think are foreign substances. Lymphocytes are the messengers that summon the troops of the immune system into action, which causes the formation of chemicals called *cytokines*. Cytokines are the "generals" of the immune army; they give orders to other types of immune cells that cause the inflammatory response. In the case of rheumatoid arthritis and other autoimmune diseases, the lymphocytes and cytokines overreact by summoning an entire platoon of immune cells, when all they really need are "a few good men." So, instead of simply eradicating the enemy, they start fighting among themselves and tearing up the landscape in the process.

There are several other diseases that fit into the category of autoimmune arthritis; there are even other disorders such as *Lyme disease* that can cause similar arthritic-like symptoms. Conventional treatments are similar for rheumatoid arthritis and all of the following types of autoimmune arthritis.

- *Ankylosing spondylitis.* A condition caused by an autoimmune attack on the joints of the spinal column. It affects about 300,000 Americans, striking twice as many men as women. Ankylosing spondylitis doesn't usually become severe enough to be completely debilitating, but in rare severe cases, joints may fuse together. It does cause chronic inflammation, which can lead to painful *sciatica* (irritation of the sciatic nerves that run down the legs) or *spinal stenosis* (where the spinal canal closes in on the nerves of the back, causing pain). Numbness, pain, and weakness in the legs also can occur. The main symptom of ankylosing spondylitis is lower back stiffness and pain, especially in the morning, that persists for more than three months. A genetic link has been found to this type of arthritis, and it often strikes people who have inflammatory bowel disease (IBD).

- *Lupus.* Also known as *systemic lupus erythematosus* or SLE, a condition in which connective tissues throughout the body become inflamed. The effects of this rare autoimmune disease vary widely from person to person and can include exhaustion, achiness, nausea, joint and muscle stiffness and aches, extreme sensitivity to sunlight, kidney disease, blood disorders, hair loss, problems with mental function, susceptibility to infection, or inflammation of the heart or lungs. The first noticeable symptoms are a butterfly-shaped rash on the face, neck, and arms, along with fever, weakness, and weight loss. In most cases, the disease goes through periods of flare-ups and remissions, but never completely goes away. SLE strikes women nine times more often than it strikes men, usually when they are between the ages of twenty and fifty. People of Asian,

African, or North American Indian descent are more likely than Cau-
casians to develop SLE.

- *Gout.* An acute form of inflammatory arthritis caused by a disorder of
  uric acid metabolism. Uric acid is a normal product of the body's
  processes, but in the case of gout, uric acid crystals build up in the
  body and become lodged in the joints, and the immune system attacks
  them. Gout typically affects the smaller joints of the feet (especially the
  big toe) and hands. About 90 percent of the 1 million Americans who
  suffer from gout are males. Drinking too much alcohol, being obese,
  and having high blood pressure increases the risk of gout.

- *Psoriatic arthritis.* A condition associated with the skin disease psoriasis,
  which is also thought to be an autoimmune disease. The inflammation
  that causes the skin irritation spreads to the joints.

- *Reiter's syndrome.* A mysterious disease that affects the eyes, urinary
  tract, and joints, primarily striking young to middle-aged men.

- *Sjögren-Larsson syndrome.* An autoimmune disease that affects moisture-
  producing glands throughout the body. Severely dry mouth, eyes, and
  skin are the most prominent symptoms, and joint pain and inflammation are often involved as well.

Chronic inflammation can cause widespread damage. In rheumatoid
arthritis, the immune attack is on the joints, sometimes spreading to other
parts of the body. It tends to come and go, with periods of intense pain
and inflammation alternating with periods of remission. The disease starts
out in the *synovium,* the lining of the joint capsule that secretes viscous
synovial fluid. From there, inflammation spreads to the cartilage, bone,
muscles, tendons, and ligaments. Deformity and disability are not uncommon in those with rheumatoid arthritis.

The hand, finger, and foot joints are most commonly affected, usually
in a symmetrical pattern. If the right hand and foot are affected, for
example, the left hand and foot probably are, too. Stiffness in the affected
joints may go away in an hour after rising in the morning or may last all
day. Those with severe rheumatoid arthritis may need help with personal
hygiene, dressing, eating, and bathing.

Carpal tunnel syndrome, tenosynovitis (inflammation of the sheaths that wrap around the wrist and finger tendons), bursitis, general weakness, and anemia (abnormal blood cell counts) are common in rheumatoid arthritis sufferers. A general feeling of being unwell, muscle pain, weakness, and low-grade fever are also typical early in the course of the disease.

Affected joints become weak, and they can be injured more easily. Small *rheumatoid nodules* are found on the tendons of rheumatoid arthritis patients, and these nodules can also form in the lungs, the eyes, or on the heart muscle. These nodules aren't harmful but their presence allows physicians to diagnose rheumatoid arthritis more accurately. Inflammation around the eyes may cause tear ducts to deteriorate, leading to dry, itchy eyes. Inflammation of the blood vessels (vasculitis), of the sac that surrounds the heart (pericarditis), or of the lungs (pulmonary fibrosis) can also occur in severe rheumatoid arthritis, and can be life threatening.

As mentioned above, most people with rheumatoid arthritis have periods of intense inflammation and pain alternating with periods of improved joint health throughout their lives. In 20 percent of the cases, the condition simply disappears and does not return. It usually is treated with NSAIDs, steroids, and immunosuppressive drugs. Physical therapy usually is necessary for those with this condition, and, if the joints are deteriorated badly, replacement surgery may be needed to avoid total disability.

Complementary medical practitioners believe that diet triggers the overreaction of the immune system that ultimately destroys joint tissues. In nations that consume the Western diet, which, in large part, is composed of processed foods that are void of vital nutrients, autoimmune diseases are far more common. Regular diets of these foods coupled with the use of NSAIDs have been linked to a condition known as *leaky gut syndrome,* which is believed to be linked to rheumatoid arthritis. (See "Leaky Gut Syndrome and Rheumatoid Arthritis" on page 12.)

INFECTIOUS ARTHRITIS

There is a third category of arthritic diseases—*infectious arthritis*—caused by a bacterial, viral, or fungal infection. Because the symptoms may be similar to autoimmune arthritis, if you visit the doctor with the symptoms of autoimmune arthritis, he or she will rule out the possibility that they are being caused by bacteria. Joints can become infected by an infectious organism that travels through the bloodstream to a joint or injury. Redness, swelling, and tenderness, often coupled with fever and body aches, are characteristic of infectious arthritis. Infectious arthritis is usually treated with antibiotics.

Leaky Gut Syndrome and Rheumatoid Arthritis

Leaky gut is actually an erosion of the gastrointestinal tract that results in tiny holes in the intestinal lining. Through this breached intestinal wall, partially digested food particles, bacteria, and other toxic microorganisms are able to pass directly into the bloodstream. Because these "invaders" don't belong in the blood, the immune system is called into action to fight them, resulting in inflammation. Furthermore, some of these toxins, which closely resemble certain joint tissues, make their way to the joints. When the immune system begins its attack, it doesn't discriminate very well and wages its war against the toxins, as well as the healthy joints themselves. One result of this immune reaction is rheumatoid arthritis. When the gut is allowed to heal through a diet of nutritious nonallergenic, whole foods, rheumatoid arthritis symptoms improve. For helpful information about leaky gut and arthritis, see Chapter 4.

CHAPTER 2

Understanding the Process of Inflammation

*I*nflammation is one way in which the body reacts to injury or illness. Any area of the body—external or internal—can display an inflammatory response. External inflammation is generally the result of an injury such as a cut or a sprained ankle, often causing swelling, redness, and pain. Common causes of an internal inflammatory response include bacterial infections, allergies, and arthritis. During an asthma attack, for example, the air passages are inflamed, making it difficult to breathe. When allergies flare, inflammation may cause a runny nose, watery eyes, and perhaps an outbreak of hives. Inflammatory bowel diseases, including Crohn's disease and ulcerative colitis, are examples of internal inflammation. These conditions are characterized by inflammation of the inner surface of the large intestine, and commonly result in abdominal pain, diarrhea, and bloody stools. A fever is an example of whole-body inflammation. Arthritis causes inflammation of the joints, resulting in swelling and pain.

Exactly what happens during the inflammatory process? To illustrate, let's take the example of a sprained ankle. An ankle sprain occurs when one of the tendons that attach your lower leg muscles to your foot is overstretched abruptly. The sudden shock tears some of the fibers that make up that tendon. Immediately, hormonal messengers called *eicosanoids* send out a message to specialized immune cells to get to the injured area and begin their healing efforts. As immune system cells migrate to the area that's injured, they pull fluid along with them, causing the area to swell. The activity of the tissue repair generates heat and causes redness.

13

While inflammation is intended to be a healing process, too much inflammation can cause great harm. In the case of arthritis, uncontrolled inflammation can cause intense fluid pressure within the joint. This pressure, coupled with the free radicals produced during the inflammatory process, can destroy tissues in the area.

FREE-RADICAL DAMAGE AND INFLAMMATION

Free radicals are atoms or groups of atoms that contain at least one unpaired electron (electrons usually occur in pairs, maintaining chemical stability). When an electron is unpaired, it hooks up easily with other molecules and can cause a harmful chemical reaction. Normally present in the body in small amounts, free radicals are necessary for the production of energy and other metabolic processes. Under normal circumstances, they are neutralized by substances known as *antioxidants*. The trouble occurs when there is excessive free-radical formation. Damage to cells, tissues, and weakness to the immune system eventually can result in a host of degenerative diseases and other health conditions.

Free radicals are caused by a number of factors, including exposure to radiation and environmental pollutants such as car exhaust, smog, and others. Diet also contributes to the formation of free radicals. The body metabolizes nutrients through diet and utilizes them along with oxygen to produce energy. During this *oxidation* process, oxygen molecules containing free radicals are released, but are then neutralized. However, oxidation occurs more readily in fat molecules than in carbohydrate or protein, meaning that a high-fat diet can increase free-radical activity.

You could liken free radicals to the exhaust created by the engine of a car. In order to convert fuel into energy, cars create hazardous exhaust. In much the same way, the body creates hazardous waste when it burns fuel for energy during metabolism.

When you slice an apple and leave it exposed to the air, oxidation causes it to turn brown. If you add lemon juice to the sliced apple, it will stay crisp and white for a longer period because the vitamin C in the lemon juice acts as an antioxidant. Antioxidants in the body help keep free radicals in check, preventing them from causing significant cell damage. When inflammation is out of control, however, free radicals outnumber antioxidants and begin to destroy cells in the affected area. In addition to dietary antioxidants like vitamin C and vitamin E, there are dozens of other plant-based substances that act as antioxidants in the body—including several of the active ingredients of ginger. Many of these will be discussed later in this book.

THE EICOSANOIDS

Prostaglandins, leukotrienes, and thromboxanes are hormones known as *eicosanoids*. Unlike other kinds of hormones, which travel through the bloodstream from the glands to distant points throughout the body, eicosanoids act locally on the cells that produce them or on other cells in

Inflammation: Creating Bodies Out of Balance

Many of our modern medical conditions can be traced back to an inflammatory process that has run amok. Allergies, asthma, osteoarthritis and rheumatoid arthritis, and other autoimmune diseases, such as Crohn's disease, ulcerative colitis, and lupus all involve inflammation that is out of control. New research is investigating a possible link between the chronic inflammation and the development of heart disease and cancer.

What makes inflammation spiral out of control, causing permanent tissue damage? In the majority of instances, a body knocked out of balance by poor diet and chronic stress is to blame. Stress on the body, caused by lifestyle or diet, changes the levels of hormones called *eicosanoids*, which are important for controlling inflammation. When the balance of these hormones is thrown off and inflammation occurs, the body is set to overreact.

Modern medicine's answer for combating excess inflammation, as it is with just about every other illness, is handed out on pages torn from prescription pads. Nonsteroidal anti-inflammatory drugs (NSAIDs), such as ibuprofen, aspirin, and acetaminophen, are commonly prescribed. Steroid drugs, including cortisone (oral and injectable) are prescribed for cases of inflammation that cannot be managed with NSAIDs. You'll see, however, that NSAIDs and steroid drugs cause as many problems as they solve.

their immediate vicinity. They are created and vanish within a fraction of a second. Each type of eicosanoid carries out its own duties in the body, with a few overlapping functions:

- *Prostaglandins* modify immunity, pain responses, inflammation, body temperature, the constriction and expansion of blood vessels, the clotting of blood, and the health of the lining of the stomach, kidneys, and small intestines.

- *Leukotrienes* modify inflammation and immunity, as well as mucous secretion and muscle contraction.

- *Thromboxanes* modify blood clotting and pain responses.

There are several types of prostaglandins, several types of leukotrienes, and several types of thromboxanes, and they have balancing effects on one another. For example, there are prostaglandins and leukotrienes that cause inflammation, and others that stifle it. There are thromboxanes that encourage the clotting of blood, and others that thin the blood and prevent clotting.

Each eicosanoid also has many subtypes. For example, prostaglandin subtypes include prostaglandins A2, A3, B1, B2, E1, and E2. While one prostaglandin subtype may work to constrict blood vessels and increase inflammation, another subtype will prevent these actions from going too far.

Balance is everything when it comes to eicosanoids. Overlapping functions of eicosanoids are designed to provide a system of checks and balances. For instance, if a prostaglandin subtype that increases pain sensation is not balanced by another subtype that decreases pain, the painful sensation will worsen. By the same token, if a leukotriene that causes increased inflammation is not balanced by one that turns off the inflammatory response at the appropriate time, then that response can harm healthy tissues.

The best way to understand this balance is to divide eicosanoids into "good" and "bad" categories. The "good" eicosanoids have health-supporting, positive effects. They help do the following:

- Decrease inflammation throughout the body.

- Maintain the proper consistency of blood, making it less likely to clot.

- Improve immune system function.

- Expand the walls of blood vessels, lowering blood pressure and improving circulation.

- Protect the stomach lining from being burned by stomach acids.

- Prevent the multiplication of cancer cells.

The harmful effects of "bad" eicosanoids cause a swing in the opposite direction. They do the following:

- Encourage inflammation.

- Cause blood to thicken.

- Decrease immune system function.

- Cause blood vessel walls to constrict.

Keep in mind that all of these hormones are necessary and that when they are in perfect balance, they counteract each other to provide an optimal environment. Problems arise when an imbalance tips the scale toward the pro-inflammatory, vessel-constrictive, blood-thickening, immune-compromising eicosanoids. (See "Inflammation: Creating Bodies Out of Balance" on page 15.)

EICOSANOIDS AND ARTHRITIS

To further explain this process, take the following example. Prostaglandin E2 (PGE2) causes pain and fever. It is one of the principal targets of aspirin and NSAIDs, which inhibit the production of this pro-inflammatory eicosanoid. PGE2 plays an important role in the development of arthritis and other inflammatory diseases. (PGE2 also decreases the activity of an immune component that seeks out and kills cancer cells. Because of PGE2's effects on cancer cells, research into the possible anticancer effects of aspirin and NSAIDs is beginning to pick up steam. Because ginger extract works by the same mechanism as NSAIDs, it's possible that it can provide the same anticancer effects; see Chapter 6.)

Prostaglandin El (PGE1), on the other hand, inhibits the clumping of blood components called platelets; it also opens up constricted blood vessels and strengthens the immune system. When PGE1 and PGE2 are balanced, inflammation is controlled and blood flows freely through the blood vessels. If PGE2 is more abundant, its negative effects predominate.

Other types of prostaglandins cause blood vessels to expand and become more permeable, so that their presence at the site of inflammation brings in more fluid. Increased fluid pressure leads to increased pain and tissue damage.

There are certain leukotrienes that increase mucous secretion, and other leukotrienes that decrease it. Some leukotrienes attract unnecessarily large numbers of immune cells to the area of inflammation, strongly upgrading the inflammatory response. If too many of these leukotrienes are present, inflammation can easily get out of hand.

If there is too much of any one eicosanoid subtype and not enough of another, the body's physiological balance point shifts slightly. It appears that a number of modern lifestyle choices, such as diets of sugar-laden and processed foods, lack of exercise, and high stress levels, shift that point toward inflammation.

DIET AND INFLAMMATION

Specifically, what affects the eicosanoid balance that contributes to arthritis inflammation? Mainly diet and stress levels.

Eicosanoids are made from essential fatty acids (EFAs)—polyunsaturated fats that are necessary for optimal health. Because the body is not able to produce EFAs, they must be obtained through the diet. Therefore, the balance of "good" and "bad" eicosanoids in the body is largely determined by the kinds of fatty acids found in the foods you eat. Once fats are digested and the fatty acids pass into the bloodstream, cells throughout the body begin turning them into eicosanoids. Enzymes are the tools that cells use to build eicosanoids from the raw material of fatty acids.

Think of your cells as tiny factories that are capable of making several different products. Which product gets manufactured depends on the raw materials that are available. Say you eat a piece of fresh salmon. During the digestive process, your body liberates the omega-3 fats, one type of

EFA, contained in the fish. Omega-3 fats contain alpha-linolenic acid (ALA), which is transformed by the enzymes *delta-6 desaturase* and *delta-5 desaturase* into eicosapentaenoic acid (EPA). EPA is then transformed by *cyclooxygenase* (COX) enzymes into "good" prostaglandins, and by *lipoxygenase* enzymes into "good" leukotrienes.

Omega-3 fats, which are found in fish oils and certain vegetable oils including canola and flaxseed, have positive health effects because they serve as the raw material for "good" eicosanoids only. Specifically, these fats are a part of nutritional treatments for rheumatoid arthritis and a host of other diseases including heart disease, inflammatory bowel diseases, high blood pressure, and weakness of the immune system. A recommended dosage of 200 milligrams of EPA per day helps to ensure the production of eicosanoids that can help relieve the pain and inflammation of arthritis.

If, on the other hand, you eat a food that is rich in a polyunsaturated fat like corn oil, omega-6 fats, the other type of EFAs, are released in the body. These fats, which also are found in other vegetable oils, raw nuts, seeds, and legumes, contain linoleic acid (LA). Linoleic acid is transformed into gamma-linolenic acid (GLA) and then to dihomo-gamma-linolenic acid (DHGLA). Now the body comes to a crossroads. The DHGLA can be transformed either into "good" eicosanoids or into arachidonic acid (AA), from which "bad" eicosanoids are created.

Arachidonic acid is the raw material from which pro-inflammatory eicosanoids are made. It is considered a nonessential fatty acid because it can be produced in the body from omega-6 fats. The Western diet, which typically is high in meat and dairy products, has too much arachidonic acid and omega-6 fats from vegetable oils, and not enough omega-3s. This creates an imbalance between the raw materials for the eicosanoids that control pain and inflammation.

Arachidonic acid from meat and dairy products, as well as from the omega-6 fats, can be made into " good" or "bad" eicosanoids. How does the body decide which type of eicosanoid should be made from arachidonic acid? It depends upon the presence of certain enzymes. When an enzyme called *cyclooxygenase-2 (COX-2)* is present, pro-inflammatory prostaglandins are made. If the enzyme *5-lipoxygenase* is present, inflammatory leukotrienes are formed. When 5-lipoxygenase or COX-2 acts on EPA from omega-3 fats, they create good leukotrienes and prostaglandins, but when they act on arachidonic acid, they create harmful pro-inflammatory leukotrienes and prostaglandins.

As you will see in the next chapter, most drugs used to treat arthritis work by inhibiting COX-2 enzymes. Inhibiting COX-2 and 5-lipoxygenase stops inflammation and pain from spinning out of control. In later chapters, you'll discover how natural remedies can also can inhibit these enzymes without any negative side effects.

Reducing Arthritis Inflammation Through Diet

In his groundbreaking book *Enter the Zone* (HarperCollins Publishers, 1996), biochemist Barry Sears describes how the foods we eat can affect eicosanoid balance. The two enzymes delta-6 desaturase and delta-5 desaturase activate the essential fatty acids. First, delta-6 activates linoleic (omega-6) and alpha-linolenic (omega-3) acids. Then delta-5 acts upon these activated fatty acids to create arachidonic acid (from linoleic acid) and eicosapentaenoic acid (from alpha-linolenic acid). If active delta-5 desaturase is not abundantly present, omega-6s are channeled into forming good eicosanoids.

According to Dr. Sears, the activity of delta-5 desaturase is what determines the direction of the eicosanoid pathway. If this enzyme is very active, the balance shifts toward the formation of arachidonic acid, and, therefore, toward the production of harmful eicosanoids. So what causes the activity of delta-5? The answer is insulin—the metabolic hormone responsible for balancing blood sugar.

A diet high in refined carbohydrates and sugars and low in protein stimulates insulin production. Through the refining process, foods such as grains and sugarcane are stripped of precious fiber and oils, leaving only the carbohydrate core to be rapidly digested. This causes blood sugar levels to shoot up quickly, which, in turn, causes a surge of insulin in an effort to bring the levels back down. Simply put, refined carbohydrates and sugars overexcite the enzymes responsible for making harmful eicosanoids. The enzymes shift into glucose-powered high gear and churn out the hormones that set the stage for inflammation.

For arthritis sufferers, the ideal diet for eicosanoid balance includes plenty of low-fat protein, vegetables, whole grains, and small amounts of fresh fruit. It contains little or no refined sugars or refined grains. For optimum health, try to eat fish at least twice a week, and eliminate as many processed foods from your diet as possible, especially those made with hydrogenated vegetable oils (margarines, vegetable shortening, and many prepared packaged foods), which disrupt the important activity of delta-6. Limit the consumption of red meat. To help balance other fats, include omega-3 rich walnuts and flaxseeds in your diet. (See Chapter 4 for more information on diet.)

STRESS AND INFLAMMATION

As stated above, the delta-6 desaturase enzyme is needed to transform linoleic and alpha-linolenic acids into activated fatty acids. This is a crucial step in the synthesis of eicosanoid hormones. When the body is under stress, hormonal changes take place. Specifically, the body pumps out the hormones adrenaline and cortisol. Among other harmful bodily effects, these hormones impede the important activity of delta-6 desaturase and cause increased insulin levels. In other words, being under stress can upset the balance between "good" and "bad" eicosanoids. Taking steps to reduce stress can help correct this imbalance, thereby contributing to the reduction of pain and inflammation. (See Chapter 8 for some helpful stress-reduction techniques.)

CHAPTER 3

Conventional Medicine and Arthritis

*A*rthritis is classified as a chronic disease, which means that there isn't any known way to cure it with drugs or medical technology. It may go away without treatment, it may come and go, or it may be a constant part of everyday life, but it shares the dubious honor, along with heart disease, diabetes, cancer, asthma, and allergies, of being one of the chronic diseases on the rise in Westernized countries. Just when modern medicine conquered most life-threatening infectious diseases in the middle of the twentieth century, the problem of chronic disease began to escalate. It continues to do so at an alarming pace.

Conventional medicine's approach to defeating infectious disease involves finding the offending organism and killing it with a powerful drug or fending it off with a vaccine. This approach doesn't work with chronic diseases because there is almost never a single, isolated factor that causes chronic disease. Complex factors including diet, lifestyle, genetics, and levels of stress and physical activity all come together to produce fertile ground for a chronic disease to take hold. Reversal of all the processes that went into creating that environment in the body requires a great deal more than a "magic bullet."

During the last decade of the twentieth century, arthritis drug research and development became a major emphasis for the pharmaceutical industry. There's an enormous market for antiarthritis drugs that promises to continue growing with the aging of the baby boomers. Many who are prescribed these drugs are expected to take them for the rest of their lives. That's a lot of money in drug company coffers. This chapter will help you to sort out the hype and the facts about these drugs, so that you can make clear decisions about how your arthritis will be treated.

The drugs used to treat arthritic conditions fall into three major categories: *nonsteroidal anti-inflammatory drugs,* or NSAIDs; *corticosteroid drugs;* and *disease-modifying antirheumatic drugs,* or DMARDs. Each type of drug works to relieve inflammation and pain, but each does so by different mechanisms. Let's take a look at each class of drugs, their risks and benefits, what they are prescribed for, what other drugs they can have harmful interactions with, and what their side effects can be. In later chapters, you'll discover how natural substances can do the work many of these drugs do, with gentler action and less risk of side effects.

As you read through this chapter, keep in mind that most drugs have more than one name—a chemical (generic) name and a brand name. Acetaminophen, for example, is sold under the brand names Tylenol, Acephen, Neopap, Redutemp, Arthritis Foundation Pain Reliever, and others. If you buy a generic version, it will simply be labeled as acetaminophen. All of these drugs are the same. Because there are so many brand names for each drug discussed, they will usually be referred to by their generic names. Make sure that you know the chemical name of any drug you are taking; if you aren't sure what that name is, ask your pharmacist.

NONSTEROIDAL ANTI-INFLAMMATORY DRUGS (NSAIDS)

Nonsteroidal anti-inflammatory drugs (NSAIDs) relieve arthritis symptoms by inhibiting COX enzymes, some of which play an important role in pain and inflammation. Aspirin—the original NSAID—was used for decades before anyone knew how it worked. In 1971, British researcher John Vane was awarded the Nobel Prize for discovering that aspirin relieved inflammation and pain by inhibiting the action of COX enzymes. Since then, other drugs have been designed to have the same action. Unfortunately, the action of NSAIDs is analogous to poisoning the whole garden to kill off a single weed. The inhibition of COX enzymes ended up causing untoward side effects because not all COX enzymes produce bad eicosanoids. Some help produce good ones as well.

Aspirin and other NSAIDs are valuable remedies for *occasional* aches, pains, or inflammation related to arthritis. NSAIDs are available over the counter and in stronger versions by prescription. In 1872, the first of the NSAIDs—aspirin—became a popular remedy. Dozens of other NSAIDs have been developed since then. Because NSAIDs pose high risk to the gastrointestinal tract when used for extended periods, physicians have had to be judicious in their use for chronic diseases. In the late 1990s, drug companies developed new NSAID drugs, including celecoxib (Celebrex). In order to understand how these drugs work, you'll need some basic information about some of the physiological processes involved in inflammation and pain, and about how NSAID drugs affect them.

All of the NSAIDs work by influencing levels of hormones called eicosanoids (see Chapter 2). The three types of eicosanoids—prostaglandins, leukotrienes, and thromboxanes—act in different, but at times overlapping, ways to modify inflammation. Maintaining the proper balance of each class of eicosanoid is an important aspect of staying healthy. NSAIDs bring down fever and control pain and inflammation by affecting the formation of these locally acting hormones.

Two types of the enzyme *cyclooxygenase*, COX-1 and COX-2, turn dietary fat into the eicosanoid known as prostaglandin. COX-1 is needed to make the prostaglandins that protect the kidneys and gastrointestinal (GI) tract. COX-2 is needed to make the prostaglandins that increase

Commonly Prescribed NSAIDs

Aspirin and Other Salicylates
- choline salicylate
- diflunisal
- magnesium salicylate
- salicylsalicylic acid
- sodium salicylate
- sodium thiosalicylate

Ibuprofen and Similar Drugs
- diclofenac
- etodolac
- fenoprofen
- flurbiprofen
- indomethacin

- ketoprofen
- ketorolac
- meclofenamate sodium
- mefenamic acid
- nabumetone
- naproxen
- oxaprozin
- piroxicam
- sulindac
- tolmetin sodium

COX-2 Inhibitors
- celecoxib (Celebrex)
- valdecoxib (BEXTRA)

inflammation and pain. Another enzyme, 5-lipoxygenase, is needed to make the leukotrienes that increase inflammation.

Older NSAID drugs inhibit the action of both types of COX enzymes, which is why they are dangerous to the GI tract and kidneys. Newer COX-2 inhibitor drugs have greater specificity for the COX-2 enzymes, which, in theory, means that they pose far less danger of adverse effects. These drugs have been widely advertised as "super aspirins."

Some pain relievers combine a salicylate or acetaminophen (see page 31 for more on acetaminophen) with sleep-inducing drugs, muscle relaxants, caffeine, or diuretics. Drugs sold under the brand names Midol, Excedrin, Pamprin, Anacin, Cope, Extra-Strength Tylenol Headache Plus, Fiorinal, Esgic, Butace, Amaphen, and Lanorinal are examples. Any drug that contains NSAIDs should state the generic name of that NSAID clearly on the label.

In the early stages of arthritic disease, conventional medicine treats a stiff, painful joint caused by autoimmune attack in much the same fashion as a stiff, painful joint caused by injury or overuse. Since rheumatoid arthritis is an inflammatory disease, it makes sense to treat it with anti-inflammatory drugs. These medications are often effective at relieving the pain of osteoarthritis, despite the fact that it rarely involves inflammation. The question is, do the benefits of NSAIDs outweigh their risks?

NSAID Side Effects

When NSAIDs are used on a daily basis, as they often are in arthritis, risk of adverse effects rises dramatically. Ulcers and gastrointestinal bleeding caused by NSAIDs kill at least 10,000 people *every year* and are the reason behind at least 76,000 hospitalizations yearly. The ulcers caused by NSAIDs are especially dangerous because the painkilling action of the drug masks the discomfort they cause, which is the body's only way to warn us of early development of an ulcer. Once bleeding becomes noticeable and appears in the stools or in the form of vomit that looks like coffee grounds, the ulcer is a serious threat. As with many prescription drugs, these drugs are also dangerous to the kidneys.

Even if NSAIDs don't cause such serious problems, they can cause a more subtle condition called *leaky gut,* as mentioned in Chapter 1. The shortage of "good" eicosanoids (particularly some types of prostaglandins) causes tiny holes to erode in the intestinal wall, allowing partly digested food and toxins into the bloodstream. As soon as these sub-stances get through the intestinal wall, the immune system tags them as foreign and attacks them. If this constant stress on the immune system goes on for very long, the immune system gets confused about what to attack and when to stop.

Leaky gut sets the stage for chronic diseases such as severe allergies, asthma, and autoimmune diseases like rheumatoid arthritis. The symp-toms of these diseases are caused by an overactive immune system, one that has lost the ability to turn itself off when it should. It isn't recognized by conventional medicine, so don't be surprised if your doctor has never heard of it. If you see a naturopathic doctor or other type of complemen-tary medical professional for treatment of allergies, asthma, or rheuma-toid arthritis, he or she will likely suspect leaky gut.

If you are using salicylates, also look out for side effects such as nau-sea, upset stomach, stomach pain, heartburn, or blood in your stools. Such side effects can mean that you're developing an ulcer or gastroin-testinal bleeding and should be attended to by a physician right away. Other side effects to look out for with salicylates include rashes, hives, anemia, easy bruising and prolonged bleeding (due to their blood-thin-ning effects), and ringing in the ears (tinnitus). They have also been asso-ciated with detachment of the retina and macular degeneration, the leading cause of blindness in the United States.

Be very wary of using salicylates if you have kidney disease, and always stop taking aspirin or other salicylates a few days before any kind of surgery to avoid excessive bleeding. Taking an aspirin an hour before having an alcoholic drink raises blood alcohol levels 26 percent higher than they would go without the aspirin. If you are using anticoagulant drugs (blood thinners), carbonic-anhydrase inhibitor drugs for glaucoma, methotrexate (prescribed for rheumatoid arthritis and other autoimmune diseases), loop diuretics, or ACE inhibitors, be aware that taking aspirin or other salicylates with these drugs can cause potentially dangerous drug interactions.

If you are using ibuprofen or similar drugs frequently, be aware that nausea, vomiting, heartburn, diarrhea, constipation, gas, cramps, or bloody stools could be the result of their use. Urinary tract problems, including increased infections and frequent urination, hepatitis, and jaun-dice can be side effects of these drugs. Other possible side effects include dizziness, drowsiness, headache, fatigue, nervousness, depression, vision, weight or blood pressure changes, mineral imbalances, menstrual problems, male impotence or breast enlargement, and anemia. Stay away from these drugs if you are scheduled for surgery, or if you have kidney or liver disease, any history of GI inflammatory disease (such as inflammatory bowel disease or Crohn's disease) or ulcer, anemia, pancreatitis, eye disease, infection, or extreme sensitivity to sunlight. Ibuprofen and similar drugs can have health-threatening interactions with anticoagulant drugs, lithium, methotrexate, ACE inhibitors, beta blockers, loop diuretics, thiazide diuretics, and DMSO (a nutritional supplement, sometimes used to treat arthritis; see page 76). Always take NSAIDs with food to minimize stomach irritation.

Another downside of NSAIDs is their effect on the hormone melatonin. Melatonin is made in a tiny gland in the brain called the *pineal gland*. When night falls, melatonin is secreted to send out the message that it's time to sleep. Children, teenagers, and young adults make plenty of melatonin and their sleep quality is usually very good. As we age, melatonin secretion drops, and we have more trouble going to sleep and staying asleep. This can be compounded by NSAID use. In one study, a single dose of aspirin decreased melatonin production by up to 75 percent.

COX-2 Inhibitors: Hope or Hype?

Drug companies have developed new NSAIDs that selectively inhibit COX-2 enzymes. These COX-2 inhibitors, often called "super aspirins," including meloxicam, celecoxib, and valdecoxib, are designed to prevent the formation of proinflammatory prostaglandins without gastrointestinal side effects. As is the case with any new drug that sounds too good to be true, there is more to know about them than the drug companies may want you to know.

COX-2 inhibitors do appear to pose less danger of side effects; however, it's clear that more research is needed before this is known for certain. The COX enzymes have so many functions that it's impossible to know the ramifications of inhibiting one of them until the drug has been thoroughly tested (which it hasn't been). We know that COX-2 plays an important role in the body's ability to repair damaged tissues and in maintaining proper blood flow through the kidneys. The result of suppressing this enzyme long-term remains to be seen. There is some dispute over whether meloxicam preferentially inhibits COX-2. The other drugs in this class inhibit COX-2 much more effectively.

There has been an amazing amount of hype surrounding COX-2 inhibitors. Arthritis sufferers have gone to their doctors in droves to ask for them, thinking they will be more effective than the NSAIDs they've been taking. In its first few months on the market, celecoxib (Celebrex) became a blockbuster moneymaker for the pharmaceutical company Searle, a subsidiary of Monsanto Company. In its first week on the market, Celebrex was prescribed to 9,923 Americans. Within thirteen weeks, it had been prescribed to 2.5 million arthritis sufferers in the United States alone. (To put this in perspective, know that Viagra, the hugely popular drug for male impotence, sold 2.7 million prescriptions in the same amount of time.) Celebrex is also being considered by the FDA for the treatment of a wider variety of conditions related to pain and inflammation.

While these drugs are a step up from the original NSAIDs, they may not live up to all of the hype that has been created about them. The truth is that the COX-2 inhibitors have not been proven more effective against arthritis pain than the older NSAIDs. There's no evidence that Celebrex will relieve symptoms the other NSAIDs aren't able to relieve.

Also, the FDA has sent drug manufacturers, physicians, pharmacists, and the public a clear message that many more long-term studies are needed to determine whether these "super aspirins" are indeed safer than traditional NSAIDs. Pharmaceutical companies are required to label COX-2 inhibitors with a warning about possible adverse gastrointestinal effects. The label informs patients that they have a 1 percent chance of developing ulcers or internal bleeding within the first three to six months of treatment, and 2 to 4 percent after a year. Users are also warned that ulcers caused by these drugs, specifically Celebrex, often crop up without any warning, so they are advised to keep an eye out for signs of gastrointestinal bleeding.

On April 20, 1999, an article in the *Wall Street Journal* reported that Celebrex had been linked to eleven cases of gastrointestinal hemorrhage and ten deaths (half of which were due to gastrointestinal hemorrhage). Searle's vice president in charge of arthritis research responded to the article by stating that the drug was "performing as expected," and that many patients who experienced side effects from Celebrex had other illnesses and had been taking other drugs—any of which could have caused their negative reactions.

COX-2 inhibitors are also very expensive—at the time of this writing, they cost approximately three dollars per dose. And like any prescription drug, they carry the risk of harmful interactions with other drugs. Asthmatics and those with high blood pressure or heart conditions are at increased health risk when using COX-2 inhibitors.

Why, if these new NSAIDs affect only COX-2 enzymes, leaving the COX-1 types alone to continue making "good" eicosanoids, do these side effects still occur? For one thing, the function of the COX enzymes is not totally specific. COX-1 and COX-2 have overlapping functions, and neither is responsible for the creation of only "good" or "bad" prostaglandins. It appears that COX-2 plays a role in tissue repair and in maintaining proper blood flow through the kidneys. Blood flow through the kidneys is an important barometer for the body, helping it regulate proper blood pressure.

Research also indicates that users of Celebrex may be increasing their risk of heart attack and stroke dramatically. It appears that this drug may be implicated in suppressing the body's formation of a prostaglandin called *prostacyclin,* which thins the blood and dilates the blood vessels.

Even if these new NSAIDs were completely harmless to the GI tract, there is another very good reason for osteoarthritis patients to try to steer clear of NSAIDs in general for long-term use: These drugs interfere with the body's ability to repair cartilage. Dozens of studies published in leading medical journals have shown this to be true. Some leading researchers have good evidence that these drugs actually accelerate the progression of osteoarthritis.

It's hard to understand why a responsible healthcare professional would prescribe anti-inflammatory drugs for a joint disease that rarely involves inflammation except in advanced stages—especially when they carry such substantial risks and slow the healing of cartilage. They do relieve pain, but there are plenty of other ways to achieve this end.

Rheumatoid arthritis is a different story. Because it's primarily an inflammatory disease, NSAIDs might be a necessary evil—at least temporarily—to prevent joint damage. Not treating out-of-control inflammation is a high-risk proposition. There are natural remedies and nutritional changes that will decrease inflammation, however, and you'll find out about those in later chapters.

ACETAMINOPHEN

Acetaminophen is a painkiller and fever reducer. Best known as Tylenol, it reduces pain by affecting the transmission of pain messages through the nervous system. It's used most in osteoarthritis patients who have difficulty with NSAIDs.

Acetaminophen Side Effects

Some who have stomach troubles from NSAIDs or are allergic to aspirin are led to believe that acetaminophen is a safe alternative. But acetaminophen isn't as safe as it's made out to be due to the considerable danger it poses to the liver. Drinking alcohol, using other drugs in combination with acetaminophen, or even just using it a little bit more often than recommended can permanently damage the liver. Even the recommended doses can put considerable stress on liver function. (See Chapter 4 for tips on supporting liver health.)

Other possible adverse effects with acetaminophen include fever, hypoglycemic coma, low white blood cell count, easy bruising, and excessive bleeding. Acetaminophen can also interact dangerously with lithium, ACE inhibitors, beta blockers, and loop diuretics. If taken with barbiturates and hydantoins, or the drugs carbamazepine, rifampin, or sulfinpyrazone, the risk of severe liver damage increases dramatically.

CORTICOSTEROID DRUGS

Cortisol is a steroid hormone made in the adrenal glands. Steroid hormones, a class that also includes progesterone, DHEA, testosterone, androstenedione, and the estrogens, are made from a hormone called *pregnenolone,* which is made from cholesterol. Without cortisol, the body cannot cope with stress. Technically speaking, we can survive without cortisol in the body, but the moment any kind of stressor enters the picture—hunger, fear, illness, or any kind of strenuous physical activity—we would become very sick or die without sufficient output of cortisol.

Now, let's say you're constantly under stress, taking in caffeine, and overexercising. All of these circumstances lead to increased cortisol production. When this hormone becomes widespread, heart rate and breathing speed up, blood flow is diverted away from the digestive tract and to muscles, and stored sugars are mobilized and passed into the bloodstream, quickly raising blood sugar levels. The activity of the immune system is suppressed. In other words, too much cortisol isn't a good thing, either.

Synthetic Cortisol

In 1949, drug researchers developed synthetic versions of cortisol, such as prednisone. Synthetic cortisols are similar to natural cortisol, but they are not found in nature, and thus can be patented. Synthetic cortisol drugs are also much more potent than those made in the body, and small doses have pronounced effects and equally pronounced side effects. The medical community began using synthetic cortisols instead of natural for economic reasons (drug companies can charge more for patent drugs) and were prescribed to treat the symptoms of inflammatory diseases and allergies. It has become common practice to call all the cortisol-related hormones made by the adrenals, as well as the synthetic versions, "cortisones," but this is inaccurate. Cortisone is a specific hormone that must be converted in the body to cortisol before it is active. In this book, we refer to cortisol and related hormones, including the synthetics, as corticosteroids.

A common treatment for rheumatoid arthritis is oral (taken by mouth) synthetic cortisol, such as prednisone (Deltasone). For osteoarthritis, it is injected into affected joints to provide relief from pain and swelling. When injected into the joints, cortisone can stave off pain for up to a few months, but because the injections are very damaging to cartilage and bone, they can't be given frequently.

Synthetic corticosteroids should always be used in the smallest possible doses for as short a period of time as possible. Only natural cortisol (usually sold as either hydrocortisone, cortisol, or Cortef) should be used long term. For anyone taking corticosteroid drugs for any length of time, the book *Safe Uses of Cortisol* by William McK. Jefferies, M.D. (C.C. Thomas, 1996), should be required reading. It details how using natural cortisol in physiologic doses (those that mimic what the body would make) can be safe and effective for a wide range of problems, including a variety of types of arthritis.

Usually, low-dose corticosteroids for rheumatoid arthritis are tried if NSAIDs don't work. The next course of action is the disease-modifying antirheumatic drugs (DMARDs), discussed below. If the DMARDs don't stop the disease from progressing, patients are put on higher doses of corticosteroids.

Corticosteroid Side Effects

Soon after the synthetic oral corticosteroids prednisone and prednisolone went into widespread use, it became obvious that they were not without serious side effects. When used for more than two weeks, synthetic corti-sone drugs can cause significant weight gain, sleeplessness, water retention, mood swings, personality changes, high blood pressure, increased risk of infections, yeast infection, cataracts, glaucoma, acne, growth of facial hair in women, osteoporosis, aseptic bone necrosis (where parts of bone tissue don't get adequate blood flow and die—a very serious problem that can destroy joints permanently), diabetes, and inflammation of the pancreas (pancreatitis). Steroid drugs are a major cause of osteoporosis in women—just a few injections over a period of a year can cause steep drops in bone mineral density.

Another problem with long-term synthetic oral steroid use is dependency. If synthetic cortisones are put into the body day after day, the adrenal glands get lazy and stop making cortisone. If the drugs are stopped abruptly, symptoms of withdrawal and even death can result. Those who have had to use these drugs long term must taper their doses gradually. They are strongly encouraged to wear a medic-alert bracelet or pendant in case of an accident, because any physician who works on them will have to take special precautions. The least stress can severely injure someone who doesn't make enough cortisone. Increased vulnerability under stress lasts for up to two years after discontinuing the medication. Synthetic corticosteroid drugs can have dangerous interactions with salicylates (aspirin), antacids, and barbiturates, and the drugs isoniazid, phenytoin, and rifampin.

If you must use synthetic corticosteroid drugs, try to do so for less than two weeks at a time. Encourage your doctor to give you the smallest possible dose. In some patients, it can be used every other day rather than every day.

DISEASE-MODIFYING ANTIRHEUMATIC DRUGS (DMARDS)

DMARDs are reserved for the treatment of rheumatoid arthritis that can't be controlled with NSAIDs or low-dose oral steroid drugs. The DMARDs are also known as slow-acting rheumatic drugs because they can take anywhere from one month to one year to become effective. Methotrexate (Trexall) works the most quickly, usually in a month to six weeks; auranofin (Riduara) can take from six months to a year to become effective. Most of the other drugs in this class take from three to six months to kick in. They may be given orally or by injection.

Traditionally, DMARDs have been reserved for use only when other measures fail to control inflammation in rheumatoid arthritis, but the most recent trend is to use them earlier to prevent permanent damage. They can be effective at stopping the progression of the disease and preventing joint damage, but as soon as the DMARDs are stopped, the symptoms return. Their often severe side effects prevent 30 percent of patients who take them from continuing long enough to gain the benefits in the first place.

It isn't known exactly how some of the DMARDs work. Many are believed to jam up the cellular equipment that drives the inflammatory process. Some of the DMARDs work by shutting down certain immune system functions, interrupting the cascade of events that leads to uncontrolled inflammation.

Two newer drugs have been introduced for the treatment of rheumatoid arthritis that doesn't respond to the other DMARDs: leflunomide and etanercept. Leflunomide (Arava) is a newer DMARD that has a mode of action and side effects similar to those of methotrexate—but with-

Commonly Prescribed DMARDs

- azathioprine
- chloroquin
- etanercept (Enbrel)
- methotrexate
- gold salts/auranofin (Riduara)
- hydroxychloroquine
- leflunomide (Arava)
- sulfasalazine

out the lung toxicity associated with the latter drug. Etanercept (Enbrel) is one of the newest DMARDs, having been approved in 1998. It works by inhibiting the binding of tumor necrosis factor (TNF) to receptors. When TNF binds to receptor sites, it triggers the formation of pro-inflammatory prostaglandins and other inflammatory cells. Blocking this reaction decreases joint inflammation in between 60 and 75 percent of those who use it. Enbrel is expensive, costing $10,000 per year per patient. Both Arava and Enbrel are often given in combination with methotrexate.

All of these medications are dangerous on their own, but can become even more so when taken with other drugs. Anyone using them must work in close communication with his or her rheumatologist and should not put any drug—over the counter, recreational, or prescription—into his or her body that hasn't been checked out with the physician first.

A decision to use any of the DMARDs is a difficult one. Their side effects can be devastating, and they don't work for every rheumatoid arthritis patient. In those patients who do respond to these drugs, relief from their disease might make the side effects worthwhile. But it's important to give natural approaches a try before resorting to such powerful medications, as soon as the disease is diagnosed. With the right diet and supplements, rheumatoid arthritis sufferers can often either postpone or avoid the need for these drugs.

DMARD Side Effects

Here are some of the side effects that may occur with the use of a number of these medications:

Auranofin (oral or injected gold salts): Diarrhea; liver damage; jaundice; skin rash; sores in mouth and on tongue; nausea; vomiting; stomach cramps; headache; partial or complete loss of hair; cough; shortness of breath; drug-induced pneumonia or lung damage; blood cell and bone marrow toxicity, leading to fatigue, sore throat, and abnormal bleeding or bruising; pain, numbness, and weakness in arms and legs (peripheral neuritis). Side effects from this drug can surface months after the drug is discontinued.

Azathioprine: Increased risk of infection; increased risk of cancer; suppression of immune cell formation in bone marrow; rash; vomiting; diarrhea; sores in mouth and on lips; liver damage; jaundice; drug-induced pneumonia.

Enbrel (etanercept): Swelling and irritation at the injection site (which in early studies occurred in 37 percent of patients); dramatic increase in risk of infection (35 percent of patients in the clinical trials developed upper respiratory and sinus infections); serious infections, including bronchitis, infectious arthritis, wound infections, pneumonia, and sepsis (a deadly infection in the bloodstream); stifling of the action of an anticancer arm of the immune system, which may lead to increased risk of cancer.

Hydroxychloroquine: Light-headedness; blue-black skin, mouth, or fingernail discoloration (with long-term use); nausea; vomiting; stomach cramps; diarrhea; hair loss or loss of hair color; headache; visual blurring; serious damage to corneas and retinas of eyes; severe depression of immune cell formation in the bone marrow; heart muscle damage; ringing in ears or hearing loss.

Methotrexate: Ulcers and bleeding in the mouth and throat; vomiting; intestinal cramping; bloody or non-bloody diarrhea; painful urination; bloody urine; reduced resistance to infection; severe depression of immune cell formation in the bone marrow; kidney, liver, and lung damage; loss of hair.

ANTIBIOTICS FOR ARTHRITIS

Since the 1930s, some arthritis experts have tried to prove that most cases of rheumatoid arthritis are caused by bacteria. Successful cures have been achieved in small studies where antibiotics were given to rheumatoid arthritis patients. The research in this area is definitely intriguing, but hasn't been consistently supportive of this theory.

Antibiotic therapy for rheumatoid arthritis is still in its experimental stages. It isn't likely that your doctor will recommend it to you until a lot more research has been done. This theory has resurfaced and been disproved so many times and the risks that accompany chronic antibiotic use are so serious that the likelihood of antibiotics becoming conventional therapy for rheumatoid arthritis is small.

SURGERY FOR ARTHRITIS

When a joint ravaged by osteoarthritis or rheumatoid arthritis loses its mobility or causes uncontrollable pain, surgery is often recommended. The type of surgery you have will depend on which joint is to be repaired and what kind of damage has been done to that joint.

The decision to have surgery is a major one. Be sure you have a second opinion before agreeing to it and, if at all possible, have outpatient surgery to avoid a hospital stay. Hospitals are not safe places for sick people. They are crawling with antibiotic-resistant infections, and misprescribed drugs kill tens of thousands of hospital patients every year. Going under general anesthesia is a risky proposition. Being in the hospital and the fear of going under the knife can be stressful all by themselves, not to mention the actual stress your body goes through while you're having the operation and starting your recovery.

Arthroscopy

In this type of surgery, the surgeon uses a very thin tube—an arthroscope—with a tiny light and camera at its tip. It's inserted through a small incision near the joint and allows the surgeon to have a look around to see how much damage has been done. A tool can be threaded through the arthroscope to cut away loose cartilage or to smooth down roughened joint surfaces. Recovery is quick and usually no hospital stay is needed.

Osteotomy

In osteoarthritis, bone can grow irregularly or can become misshapen. Osteotomy is the surgical removal of deformed bone to improve the function of a joint.

Resection

Resection involves the removal of part or all of one of the small bones in the foot, wrist, elbow, or thumb when osteoarthritis causes severe deformity or pain.

Arthrodesis

When joints are beyond repair, the two halves can be fused together. The joint is no longer movable but becomes much less painful and more stable. Usually this surgery is done on the joints of the thumb, ankles, wrists, or fingers. In some instances of arthritis in the backbone, vertebrae are fused together.

Arthroplasty

Also known as joint replacement, arthroplasty is a last resort for arthritic hips, knees, shoulders, elbows, ankles, and knuckles. The surgeons replace the degenerated joint with an artificial one. This type of surgery is serious and entails at least a week's hospital stay and outpatient physical therapy, but in many cases can rescue patients with advanced arthritis from becoming invalids. It's a good thing these procedures exist and are relatively safe and effective, but all possible measures should be taken to prevent the disease from progressing this far. The older and feebler the patient is, the greater the risks involved with arthroplasty.

Synovectomy

This surgery involves the removal of diseased synovial tissues from joints of rheumatoid arthritis patients. The synovium does grow back, and the procedure often needs to be repeated within a few years' time. This procedure is done with an arthroscope.

Caring for Yourself Before and After Arthritis Surgery

If you do have to go to the hospital for your surgery, be sure to prepare yourself adequately. Here are some guidelines for you to follow if you will be having inpatient surgery. You should advise your doctor of any supplement, vitamin, or drug you are taking prior to surgery.

- **Support your liver**, which will have to process a great many drugs during your surgery and your recovery. The herb milk thistle (use as directed on the container), alpha lipoic acid (200 mg three times a day with meals), and N-acetyl-cysteine (500 mg three times a day with meals) all promote the health of the liver. Use these nutrients for one week prior to surgery and for two weeks after surgery. If you are diabetic, be aware that alpha lipoic acid can cause blood sugar levels to drop; start out with 50 mg twice a day and build up slowly, and let your physician know you are using it. Also, get plenty of fiber in your diet to keep your bowels moving—constipation interferes with good liver function.

- **Improve your immune system function** before going into the hospital. Vitamin A (not its precursor, beta-carotene) is the best choice for improving immune function. Take 15,000 IU a day for the week before surgery, 50,000 IU a day for the two days before, and 15,000 IU for about ten days following. If you are pregnant, don't take more than 15,000 IU a day. Also take 1,000–2,000 mg of vitamin C, 200 mcg of selenium, and 15 mg of zinc—in addition to your regular daily supplements.

- **Discontinue use of salicylates or other NSAIDs,** which thin the blood, at least one week before surgery. You should be able to continue taking 400 IU a day of vitamin E, which is a mild blood thinner. Check with your doctor to make sure.

- **Take bioflavonoid antioxidants,** such as green tea extract or grapeseed extract after surgery to speed healing. Follow the instructions on the container. The amino acid glutamine helps your body destress and detoxify, and aids in good digestion. Use 500 mg twice a day, for a total of 1,000 mg, between meals, for one week before and two weeks after your surgery.

- **Learn relaxation techniques** to help you cope with stress and pain before, during, and after your hospital stay. See Chapter 8 for some helpful relaxation techniques.

CONVENTIONAL MEDICINE VERSUS NATURAL MEDICINE

If you read the Arthritis Association's extensive patient literature, you'll find it adheres to conventional medical approaches almost exclusively. It devotes a few passages here and there to "unproven remedies," basically advising readers to steer clear of supplements and natural treatments. Their reasoning is that even if one of these so-called unproven remedies is harmless, it can cause damage to the body simply because it does not stop the destruction of joint tissues. They warn against some supplements because they have potential side effects and emphasize the fact that not as much research has been done on natural remedies as has been done on prescription drugs. However, conventional medicine practitioners neglect to mention some key points in their dismissal of natural approaches.

Of all the drugs used to treat arthritis, not a single one is free of the potential for side effects—and those caused by drugs are far more serious than those caused by natural remedies. This fact is glaringly obvious to anyone who reads the Arthritis Association's literature about the drugs commonly used to treat arthritis. They also don't mention the new "fast-track" approval system for prescription drugs, which allows drugs to go on the market after minimal testing, or the fact that, according to the *New*

England Journal of Medicine, prescription drug errors and side effects kill at least 140,000 Americans a year. If any nutritional supplement manufacturer had that kind of track record, you can bet the FDA would close them down pretty quickly.

What you don't often hear is that some conventional treatments used for osteoarthritis could cause the disease to progress more rapidly than it would were it not treated at all. This is, of course, not mentioned in the Arthritis Association's consumer information warnings. Instead, they mention that supplements could be harmful if they don't actually control or reverse the disease. When you also consider that conventional treatments are not effective for everyone, this particular argument against natural medicine for arthritis loses its clout.

Drugs and conventional medical intervention may not always be the answer for arthritis recovery. It is known that many of the biochemical changes that go on in joints affected by osteoarthritis are geared toward repairing damaged tissues and restoring the function of those joints. This is good evidence that the best we can do for osteoarthritis may be to give the body the raw materials it needs to do this job on its own—with the right diet and supplements—rather than loading it up with drugs. Amazingly, in a study that traced the natural progression of osteoarthritis without medical treatment, researchers discovered that nearly half of the patients who had advanced hip arthritis recovered without any medical intervention. Their bodies were able to reverse the course of the disease.

In the case of rheumatoid arthritis, which can pose the threat of permanent joint deformity, the use of medications and surgery may be necessary to deal with episodes of severe inflammation. You'll find, however, that there are dietary changes, supplements, and natural remedies that can make a difference, even when they are used along with conventional treatments.

Why Natural Is Safer than Synthetic

It's quite rare that anyone suffers any type of side effects from supplements or natural remedies. This is because they are substances that occur in nature that work in harmony with the body's complex systems. Drugs, which are natural molecules altered in laboratories, are designed to potently affect a single variable in one of those systems. The slightest alteration in the structure of a natural molecule can create a substance with a much more powerful effect on human physiology. Increased power of action means increased risk of adverse effects.

Drug manufacturers are usually aiming for the greatest possible specificity. When a drug has *specificity*, it works to alter a single biochemical reaction in the body, without affecting other reactions. The problem with this is twofold. On the one hand, if a single system is affected—if the "magic bullet" hits its mark exactly—it creates an imbalance with other systems that should be integrated with it. This imbalance could cause drug side effects.

Also, it rarely happens that a drug is absolutely specific. What more often causes drug side effects is a lack of specificity. If the "magic bullet" doesn't exactly strike its mark, it affects not only the system it's aimed at, but other interdependent ones as well. For example: one class of drugs is designed to relieve joint inflammation by inhibiting the production of certain biochemicals. These substances belong to a larger class of biochemicals, some of which are important for other body functions. The drugs aren't specific enough to inhibit only those that cause inflammation and instead inhibit the whole class, causing adverse effects. This is the case with the most commonly prescribed drugs for arthritis, NSAIDs.

You may have found yourself caught in this crossfire yourself as you have tried to make the best choices for your own health. Making your task harder, politics and economic issues surrounding pharmaceutical companies, the medical industry, and physician education have considerable influence on what information reaches physicians and the public. Money from pharmaceutical interests funds much of the medical research done in this country. Pharmaceutical companies have little desire to pay for research on nutritional supplements. Natural substances can't be patented, and so drug companies can't name their prices and make huge profits the way they can by altering natural substances and patenting them for use as drugs.

This is not to say that there aren't unethical supplement manufacturers out there who are trying to sell you something worthless. That's why it's so important to find information you can trust, and to be able to talk with your doctor about whether a natural remedy could work for you. There are some wonderful manufacturers of nutritional supplements who maintain rigorous standards of quality based on excellent research. It's simply a matter of separating the wheat from the chaff.

CHAPTER 4

Eating to Combat Arthritis and Promote Good Health

*M*any people have asked some version of this question: "Why should I think that my diet has anything to do with my arthritis, when I've eaten this way all my life and didn't have arthritis until now?" A youthful body can usually handle a diet of processed foods, because its digestive and cleansing mechanisms are in peak condition. As you age, those mechanisms don't function as well and need a little more care and attention. A suboptimal diet also has cumulative effects over a lifetime, so that the adverse effects may not show up until your fifties or sixties.

But to eat right and help combat the symptoms of arthritis, you do not have to ride the wave of any fad, but instead simply eat a diet that is natural, uncomplicated, and based on common sense.

In this chapter, you will learn how to eat a diet that will decrease the amount of inflammation in your body. Although not all arthritis involves uncontrolled inflammation in the joints, a diet designed to help prevent inflammation from setting in promotes health in many ways. Inflammation is being linked to a wide variety of conditions besides autoimmune disorders—from heart disease to Alzheimer's disease to cancer. We don't know if it causes disease or if it's an effect of disease, but either way it makes sense to eat a diet that will help keep potentially harmful inflammation from spinning out of control.

The dietary approaches to osteoarthritis and rheumatoid arthritis overlap in many respects. Doing all you can to support your digestive tract and liver is the foundation for any arthritis-busting diet. This chapter will show you the essentials on how these organs work, what can go wrong there, and about how your joint health depends upon their proper functioning. And, in addition to adding whole foods to your diet, you will learn the importance of drinking enough water, eating less food in general, protecting your body from leaky gut and food allergies, and how fasting can help reduce inflammation. If you follow all of the dietary guidelines in this chapter, you will take the first step toward reducing inflammation and easing your arthritis. Then, by adding some of the supplements and natural remedies described in later chapters, you can experience even more profound results.

THE DIETARY CONNECTION TO CHRONIC DISEASE

Chronic diseases such as arthritis, heart disease, diabetes, cancer, osteoporosis, allergies, asthma, and autoimmune disease are affecting more people in modernized nations than ever before. The medical research community has put much effort into pinpointing the causes of these diseases. They've come up with a wide variety of possible causes: genetic predisposition, too much fat in the diet, certain kinds of fat in the diet, certain chemicals in the environment, viruses, too much sugar, not enough calcium, and countless others. If you're trying your best to prevent or heal chronic disease, you may often find yourself confused by conflicting advice based on the latest theories.

I believe one of the most important answers to this state of affairs is a simple one: that a diet of refined, processed foods, rather than fresh, whole foods, plays a major role in the increase in chronic diseases. Refined and processed foods include canned and frozen food, refined white flour products (breads, bagels, baked goods, pasta), chips, sweets, meats such as bologna and hot dogs, and all the rest of those foods lining the grocery store shelves that are long on sugary, salty, or fatty taste and short on nutrition.

Eating primarily whole foods is not an extreme diet although it may seem so at first if you're accustomed to the standard American diet (SAD), where ketchup and french fries are considered vegetables and where most food and drink have been stripped of nutrients and are full of added sugar, salt, flavorings such as MSG, and preservatives. Eating in a way that supports joint health provides the right environment in your body for any arthritis treatment plan to be as effective as possible—whether you decide to use conventional medical approaches, natural approaches, or a combination of the two.

In osteoarthritis, the right diet supports the repair of damaged cartilage. Taking steps to support the function of your digestive and cleansing organs will help you to get the full value of foods and supplements that support joint health. It's also important for those with osteoarthritis to find a diet that will help drop excess pounds. Obesity is a major contributing factor in this form of arthritis, because it increases stress on the joints.

A diet to slow the progression of rheumatoid arthritis is designed to keep inflammation in check. The concepts of toxicity and biochemical individuality are especially significant in autoimmune arthritic diseases such as rheumatoid arthritis and lupus. (See "Limit Your Exposure to Toxins" on page 46.) Some people are more susceptible to these disorders than others. It could be genetics, stress, hormone imbalances, overexposure to *endo-* or *exotoxins,* or a combination that triggers an overblown immune response.

Support Your Digestive System

Your digestive system creates an interface between your body and the environment. The role of the group of organs in your digestive system— also known as the gastrointestinal (GI) tract—is to break down what you eat and drink into its most basic molecular components and to pick and choose what passes through its walls into the bloodstream.

Whatever isn't absorbed has to be disposed of, and this is another part of the job done by the digestive and cleansing organs. Any exotoxins that do get absorbed, along with the endotoxins created inside the body, are—ideally—filtered out of body fluids and disposed of by the liver and kidneys. In ancient healing practices, such as Chinese and Indian (Ayurvedic) medicine, supporting the function of the kidneys and liver is part of healing many illnesses. These organs are among our best allies in the fight against disease, and a healthy, toxin-free diet is the best way to keep your kidneys and liver in good working order. One of the shortcomings of modern drug-based medicine is that damage to the kidneys and liver are common side effects of even the safest drugs.

Let's take a whirlwind tour through your digestive tract, so that you have a good basic understanding of how everything works. This will help you to understand what can go wrong.

Limit Your Exposure to Toxins

A toxin is any substance that can do damage to living tissue. Some toxins, called *exotoxins* (*exo* = exterior), come into the body from outside. Examples of exotoxins are prescription drugs, chemicals found in the environment, artificial food additives, and preservatives. Even some of the foods we think of as health-promoting, such as milk, tomatoes, soybeans, or wheat, contain natural toxins that some people react to unfavorably.

Other types of toxins, called *endotoxins* (*endo* = interior), are formed within the body in the natural course of its day-to-day functions. Inflammation and other immune system activities produce toxins that can kill healthy cells. Potentially toxic substances are manufactured by unfriendly bacteria of yeasts that live in the body. A healthy body can easily handle these types of toxins in small amounts.

Toxicity isn't so much about the substance itself, but about the way it interacts with a person's body. Something that is quite toxic to one person can be harmless to another. For example, in a person with a peanut allergy, the minutest bit of peanut protein can kill. The rest of us can eat a peanut butter and jelly sandwich without a second thought. Even poisonous chemicals such as pesticides and herbicides are less toxic to some people than they are to others.

Most of us have a relative who's been smoking and drinking since his teens and who is still going strong into his eighties. Another example of this concept—which science refers to as biochemical individuality—is the fact that while one person may suffer debilitating side effects from a drug, another person can take it for years without any problem.

Certain people have bad reactions to toxins when they accumulate beyond what the body can process. Some people can handle more than others. A complex interplay of genetics and one's past and present habits create these differences. The capacity of the digestive organs and the organs that neutralize toxins varies from person to person. During a person's lifespan, subtle changes in the body, diet, or environment can cause new sensitivities to crop up; along the same lines, reactivity to toxins can fade with time.

The Stomach

The stomach's job is to break down food as completely as possible, so that when it goes into the small intestine, it's ready to be absorbed into the bloodstream and distributed throughout the body. It does so by secreting *hydrochloric acid* (HCl) and a protein-digesting enzyme called *pepsin,* and mixing them into the food with strong contractions. Another ring of muscle separates the stomach from the small intestine. When the acidity of the stomach contents now called *chyme* reaches a certain level, that muscle gets the signal to relax. The chyme is then passed in small squirts into the small intestines.

The Small Intestine

Near the mouth of the small intestine lies the pancreas. This small organ secretes enzymes into the chyme to further digest proteins, carbohydrates, and fats. These enzymes dismantle large food molecules, reducing them to their most basic elements, the *macronutrients.* It is these elements—fatty acids (from fats), sugars (from carbohydrates), and amino acids (from proteins)—that we finally absorb into the bloodstream and distribute to where they are needed. Vitamins, minerals, and other micronutrients are also liberated and absorbed during this part of digestion.

The small intestine is a complex organ, an excellent example of multi-tasking—it's a digestive organ and an immune system organ rolled into one. Its twists and turns are lined with what looks like a microscopic shag carpet. Tiny nubs called *villi* cover its surface, increasing the surface area through which nutrients can be absorbed. Each villus contains a network of *capillaries.* Capillaries are blood vessels with walls that are a single cell thick, through which nutrients pass to be carried away to wherever they are needed. The small intestine is also lined with a vast array of immune cells, designed to distinguish between what should and should not be absorbed. These immune cells bar entry to whatever they perceive to be potentially toxic.

The Liver

The liver is the largest solid organ in the body, weighing in at about five pounds. Think of the liver as the body's internal sewage treatment plant, filtering wastes and toxins out of the bloodstream and disposing of them.

Drugs, alcohol, toxic chemicals, hormones, allergens, used immune cells, and infectious microbes are all processed by the liver. Aside from its detoxification function, the liver also functions in the production of bile (which is needed for the digestion of fats in the small intestine), cholesterol, and blood-clotting factors. It provides storage space for carbohydrates, vitamins, and iron, and converts many vitamins into their active, biologically useful forms.

Let's say you're rushed for dinner one night and have a fast-food hamburger, soda, and fries. The drugs given to the cattle, the preservatives in the roll, the caffeine in the soda, and the pesticide residues on the french fries are absorbed into the bloodstream from the intestines. From there, they are transported directly to the liver through the portal vein. When the digestive tract is working well, and the toxic load isn't too great, the liver can neutralize and dispose of these toxins. If you eat fast food every day, however, the liver can become overworked. The drugs and pesticides may end up sitting permanently in your fat cells, and the caffeine and preservatives may sit in the bloodstream longer. An overburdened liver is especially common among those who frequently use over-the-counter and prescription drugs, alcohol, and caffeine. If this happens, toxicity builds up and contributes to chronic disease. As we age, the liver's cleansing powers decrease. This is one reason why older people are at higher risk for adverse effects from drugs: the liver doesn't clear substances from the bloodstream as quickly, so the drug stays in the system longer.

As the liver neutralizes toxins twenty-four hours a day, seven days a week, it creates loads of free radicals in the process. An important antioxidant, called *glutathione,* is made in the liver to protect it from free-radical damage. A shortage of glutathione can spell trouble for the liver, especially when toxic load is high. The standard American diet falls far short of supplying adequate raw materials to make glutathione. Glutathione can't be absorbed through the GI tract, and so it doesn't help to supplement the diet with this antioxidant.

Supporting the health of the liver means cutting way back on over-the-counter drugs and alcohol, and eating an organic whole-foods diet (see page 53). Given the opportunity, the liver can do an amazing repair job on itself—even after years of abuse. Supplements that support the liver include alpha lipoic acid and the herb milk thistle. Foods rich in sulfur, such as eggs, garlic, asparagus, and onions, boost glutathione levels in the liver, helping to protect it as it does its important work. For additional sulfur, always a good idea for an overworked liver, you can use MSM (methylsulfonylmethane) or glucosamine sulfate (which has the added bonus of repairing cartilage).

The Large Intestine

As wastes passes into the large intestine (usually referred to as the colon) from the small intestine, the body tries to conserve water and minerals by reabsorbing them through the colon walls. More water and minerals are reabsorbed when you're dehydrated and depleted of minerals. This means that stools get hard and difficult to pass—good reasons for you to drink plenty of water and take a complete mineral supplement. (See "Relieve Constipation" on page 50.)

Our large intestine actually houses an entire ecosystem, including *probiotics* (friendly bacteria), yeasts, and less friendly *putrefactive* bacteria. We have a symbiotic relationship with probiotics, which means that we help them and they help us. They have a place to live and plenty to eat—they dine on undigested bits of food and fiber—and they do some valuable work for us in return. Probiotics manufacture B vitamins and vitamin K, which are absorbed into the body through the colon walls. They produce natural antibiotic substances that keep putrefactive bacteria such as *E. coli,* salmonella, and clostridium at bay, and help to get rid of chemical toxins. Probiotics also make a substance that prevents the growth of cancer cells in the colon.

Whenever something goes wrong in your digestive tract, it's a sign that things are out of balance. Rather than opting for a quick fix with symptom-suppressing medication, look to natural remedies and dietary changes to get relief.

Tips for Eating Well to Support Your Digestive System

Many of the chronic illnesses that are becoming so common, including arthritis, can be traced back to imbalances in the digestive system, whether the stomach, small intestine, or large intestine. These imbalances are directly related to the consumption of the processed-food, nutrient-depleted standard American diet. Conventional medicine has not yet recognized the importance of a balanced digestive system, making the above diseases difficult for conventional doctors to diagnose or treat.

Relieve Constipation

If you don't have at least one bowel movement a day, you should take steps to relieve constipation. When your bowels don't move regularly, toxins meant to be eliminated quickly sit too long in the colon and can be reabsorbed into the bloodstream, thereby causing inflammation. Other bowel toxins, when allowed to sit too long, are transformed into carcinogens by naturally occurring chemicals in the large intestine. Constipation can also lead to hemorrhoids (varicose veins in the anus) and diverticulosis (the forming of pouches in the intestines where food can get trapped and cause dangerous infections). Both are the result of straining to evacuate the bowels.

Food allergies, leaky gut, and yeast overgrowth all contribute to the problem of constipation. (These three problems are interrelated and often exist in the same people.) But if you switch to a whole-foods diet, drink six to eight glasses of water a day, and treat food allergies and yeast overgrowth, it's likely that your constipation will disappear. If it doesn't, you can try a fiber supplement. Psyllium husk is a cheap and effective source of fiber available at your local health food store. Mix one to three teaspoons of psyllium in a 6- to 8-ounce glass of water or juice and drink it immediately. Follow it with another glass of water. If you tend to have problems with intestinal gas, start with a teaspoon or less and build up slowly.

You can support your digestive function with the right diet, but if you've been eating the standard American diet for some time, or if you have chronic indigestion or irritable bowel syndrome, you'll need a little extra help to get back on track. Following are a list of tips that can help boost the strength of your digestive tract:

- Take a digestive enzyme and betaine HCl (hydrochloric acid) supplement at each meal. Make sure it contains protein, fat, and carbohydrate-digesting enzymes—protease, lipase, and amylase, respectively.

- Take a refrigerated probiotic supplement between meals to ensure that you have adequate friendly bacteria, especially if you have recently had to take antibiotics, which indiscriminately kill off good and bad bacteria.

• Get plenty of fiber in your diet by eating plenty of whole foods. Fiber is found in unprocessed fruits and vegetables, whole grains, nuts, and seeds.

Do You Need Supplemental Digestive Enzymes?

If you tend to have gas and lower abdominal bloating after you eat, try using supplemental digestive enzymes. Gas is formed when undigested food is fermented by bacteria in the colon. If you don't make enough stomach acid and digestive enzymes, a lot of digestion remains to be done in the colon, which means a lot of uncomfortable and potentially embarrassing gas will form. In the case of lactose intolerance, the carbohydrates in milk aren't digested at all, and when they hit the colon they cause gas, bloating, and diarrhea.

Intestinal gas is another problem that will probably disappear when you correct your diet by eating plenty of raw and whole foods. Fresh papaya and pineapple are both rich in protein-digesting enzymes. You can buy these enzymes in supplement form to take after meals. A full-spectrum enzyme supplement, containing amylase (for carbohydrate digestion), lipase (for fat digestion), protease (for protein digestion), and lactase (for lactose digestion), will give you better digestive support. Pineapple enzyme, or bromelain, also happens to be a potent anti-inflammatory. You'll find out more about this use for bromelain in Chapter 5.

Eat a Whole-Foods Diet

Refinement and processing of foods strips them of their nutritional value. Refined foods tend to have strong, even addictive, tastes compared to vegetables, fruits, and whole grains, but they are appetizing only because of all the sugar, salt, oils, and other additives and flavorings they contain. Food manufacturers sometimes add vitamins and minerals to their products, but this hardly makes them equal in nutritional value to whole foods.

Whole foods are those that have undergone minimal or no processing, that are as close as possible to their natural state. The staples of a whole-foods diet are fresh vegetables, whole grains, legumes (beans), fruit, raw nuts and seeds, and occasional servings of organic meats, fish, poultry, and dairy products. Herbs, spices, and healthy oils add flavor and variety.

Contrary to popular belief, this kind of diet can be delicious and satisfying. Our taste buds have grown accustomed to the powerful and addictive tastes of sugar, salt, and other artificial flavorings. Whole foods have more delicate flavors that we need to adjust to if we've been eating primarily refined foods. Once you make the shift, though, you'll feel so much better that you'll never want to go back.

A whole-foods diet is one of the surest ways to keep your body youthful, energetic, slim, and free of disease. Of course, it's hard for some people to imagine eating nothing but whole foods. Even if you can't go all the way with it, try to replace processed foods with whole foods whenever you can—even small changes in your diet can be beneficial. There are a few non-negotiables here, however.

Kick Your Sugar Habit

Americans eat approximately 133 pounds of sugar a year. Sugar—including white and brown varieties, fructose (fruit sugar), maple syrup, and honey—all cause blood sugar levels to fluctuate. When you eat a sugary snack, your blood sugar rises way above normal. High blood sugar is harmful to the body in many ways, and so the pancreas comes to the rescue, pumping out plenty of insulin. Insulin's job is to pull sugar out of the blood and store it in the cells. It does its job so well that blood sugar levels plummet. You then suffer from the shakes, foggy thinking, and fatigue, and soon you're craving another dose of refined sugar.

Cutting way down on sugar and refined grains (white flour, pasta, white rice) is an important aspect of an anti-inflammatory diet. Processed food diets, especially those high in refined grains and sugar, are directly linked to the insulin and blood sugar imbalances that lead to adult-onset (type 2) diabetes. Adult-onset diabetics have high blood sugar and high insulin levels, both of which are devastating to the body. One of the ways in which high insulin levels cause damage is by dramatically increasing the production of pro-inflammatory eicosanoids.

Sugar also depletes your body of B vitamins and the minerals magnesium, chromium, and copper. It suppresses your immune system, damages your kidneys, worsens allergies, and raises blood fats (cholesterol and triglycerides). It's true that some forms of sugar are less harmful than others—honey and maple sugar are less refined, and so have a less intense effect—but they'll put you on the sugar addiction treadmill just as the others do. Your best bet is to break your sugar habit entirely and to reserve sweets for the most special of occasions.

Bypass the Bread and Pass on the Pasta

Flour—especially white flour—has virtually the same effect on the body as sugar does. When wheat is stripped of its husk and oils and made into flour, it's called a refined carbohydrate and it essentially becomes sugar. It has virtually no nutritional value and causes blood sugar to swing rapidly up and down. Making these foods your mainstay is only slightly healthier than living on sweets.

If you can't live without bread, find a variety made with the whole grain. They should say "whole grain" on the label, not just "whole wheat." Corn tortillas are another healthful alternative to bread. Use whole grains—brown rice, quinoa, barley, polenta, and millet—instead of pasta. They cook up quickly and taste great with vegetables.

Make Raw Foods a Part of Your Daily Diet

Raw foods contain enzymes that aid digestion and absorption of nutrients, whereas cooking shuts off all enzyme activity and destroys water-soluble vitamins such as vitamin C. Unfortunately, most people eat virtually no raw food. Fresh fruit at breakfast and a green salad with dinner are excellent ways to add raw foods to your diet. Buy locally grown produce whenever you can; when it sits for long periods in trucks and on supermarket shelves, levels of enzymes and vitamins decrease.

Go Organic

One of the best ways to ensure you are getting the healthiest whole foods in your diet is to buy organic meat, grains, dairy products, eggs, and produce. When you sit down to a meal, you don't intend to eat polychlorinated biphenyls (PCBs), phthalates, bovine growth hormones, altered fruit and vegetable genes, organochlorine pesticides, antibiotics, or insecticides. If you aren't eating organic foods, it's a safe bet these toxins are a part of your daily diet. If you're eating processed foods, you're probably swallowing monosodium glutamate (MSG), aspartame, tartrazine, sodium benzoate, sodium nitrite, and a host of other additives and preservatives with your meals.

The chemicals listed above have been linked with a wide variety of chronic diseases, including cancer, liver disease, brain disease, autoimmune diseases, such as rheumatoid arthritis, and diseases of the reproductive tract. Despite the food and chemical industries' efforts to minimize public knowledge of the harm these toxic substances can do, more people than ever before are taking the initiative to find out the truth—and they're buying organic.

Most cattle and poultry in North America are raised in crowded conditions and fed a diet that is far from optimal. As a result, they are riddled with diseases for which they are then given antibiotics and other drugs. In addition, before they are sent to market they are fed estrogens to fatten them up. Those drugs end up in your body when you eat their meat or eggs, or drink their milk. Vegetables, fruits, and grains that are not organic are sprayed with pesticides, fungicides, chemical fertilizers, weed killers, and petrochemical-containing waxes.

The companies that make these chemicals insist that they are safe in the amounts people are exposed to. They said that about DDT, asbestos, and atrazine, too—chemicals that were finally banned when the evidence became overwhelming that they were carcinogenic and hormone-altering. When a new chemical is introduced, it goes through basic animal testing to be sure it doesn't cause birth defects or cancer. What we know now, however, is that often the harmful effects of chemical toxins don't appear until years after being exposed, or in the offspring of people or animals who have been exposed. Until there is overwhelming evidence of an approved chemical's toxicity, it can stay on the market. The evidence that chemical toxins that are used on crops are harming humans, animals, and the environment continues to grow. The interactions between different chemicals are impossible to predict, and the typical person is exposed to dozens of different ones a day, in various combinations. Your best bet is to avoid them whenever you can. Eating organic food is one way to accomplish this end.

Organic foods are raised and grown under strict guidelines. Only natural methods are used on crops to get rid of pests and to encourage plants to grow. Animals raised organically are kept in humane conditions and are fed only organic feed. Organics are more expensive, because the process of raising them is more labor-intensive, but they're definitely worth it. The number of food dollars being spent on organics has already made conventional farmers take notice: they recently tried to persuade the government to make the guidelines much more lenient. Rather than changing their mode of operations, the industry attempted to change the rules so that their present chemical-intensive practices would be considered organic! Fortunately, well-informed consumers made such uproar about these proposed changes that they didn't go into effect.

If you only switch one part of your diet to organics, make it animal foods—meat, poultry, dairy, and eggs. Some of the most dangerous toxins become concentrated in the fat of animal foods, and that's where you get the highest doses of these chemicals. One exception to this rule is fish, for which a set of organic labeling requirements hasn't been made. Eat more of the deep-water varieties such as salmon, cod, sardines, and mackerel. Tuna and swordfish have a higher level of mercury than most fish, so don't eat them more than once a week. Generally avoid bottom-feeding shellfish such as clams and oysters.

Conventional cleaning supplies, bug sprays, air fresheners, and beauty products also contain many ingredients with unknown or harmful effects on the body. It isn't necessary to find "organic" products for these purposes, but finding natural alternatives in your health food store will lower your toxic load substantially. You can also make your own cleaning supplies and insect repellents from natural ingredients. More nontoxic choices are available now that people are becoming aware of the threat of living and working in a soup of chemical fumes.

Use Healthy Oils

Three major categories of fats exist in whole foods: saturated (found in meats and dairy products), monounsaturated (found in olive, canola, avocado, and nut oils), and polyunsaturated (found in plant, seed, and soybean oils).

The saturation of a fat molecule describes the stability of that fat—its resistance to spoiling, or *oxidizing*. Oxidation is a natural process that occurs when fats are exposed to oxygen, creating free radicals, which damage cells. The more saturated the fat, the more resistant it is to oxidation. As you may recall from Chapter 2, the body uses antioxidant nutrients, such as vitamins C and E, to neutralize free radicals. If our free-radical load is high and our antioxidant intake low, the overflow of oxidation can be highly destructive to our tissues. Excess free radicals are a likely common denominator in the causes of many chronic diseases.

Pro-inflammatory and anti-inflammatory eicosanoids (see Chapter 3) are made out of the fats we consume. If there is an imbalance between certain types of fat in the diet, there tends to be an imbalance between pro- and anti-inflammatory eicosanoids. Fats found in meats and dairy products are some of the most overconsumed fats in the standard American diet. In fact, these fats are the raw material from which some of the pro-inflammatory eicosanoids are made. Fat from fish, seeds, nuts, and vegetables (yes, vegetables do contain tiny amounts of fat) are needed to make the anti-inflammatory eicosanoids. The most important fats to cut out completely are the hydrogenated oils or trans-fatty acids, found in virtually all processed foods, margarines, and vegetable shortenings.

While you are being careful to get the right kinds of fats in your diet, it is, at the same time, equally important not to become fat-phobic. You do need saturated fats, too—just not in the amounts most Americans eat them. A small amount of butter or whole milk adds a lot of flavor to foods, and if you add these fats to your diet in moderate amounts they shouldn't cause you any harm.

Polyunsaturated fats, and their close cousins, the hydrogenated fats, should be avoided. Polyunsaturated fats, such as corn oil, safflower oil, and cottonseed oil, are very unstable and oxidize easily. Heating them to high temperatures for cooking produces many free radicals.

Hydrogenated oils are the food industry's attempt to solve this problem. By bombarding unsaturated oils with hydrogen atoms, food manufacturers create fats that are more stable and resistant to spoilage. It turns out, however, that these fake fats contain trans-fatty acids that increase the risk of artery-clogging plaques and heart attacks. They are much worse for you than any saturated oil, and not much better than the rancid unsaturated oils. Virtually all processed and refined foods contain hydrogenated or "partially hydrogenated" oils.

The gold standard is monounsaturated oil. Olive oil is your best bet; it's delicious, and the extra virgin varieties are only minimally processed. Canola oil is best for baking and cooking foods that don't taste right with olive oil. These oils are only slightly less stable than saturated fats.

Eat Your Fish

Deepwater fish, such as salmon, mackerel, and cod, are loaded with heart-healthy omega-3 fats. These fats are polyunsaturated, but in their natural form (such as in fish) they do not go rancid before the fish goes bad, and they have potent anti-inflammatory effects that can benefit arthritis suffers. They can also lower cholesterol, protect against certain forms of cancer, and help to thin the blood (which helps prevent blood clots that cause heart attacks and strokes). To fully experience these benefits, enjoy baked or poached fish two to three times a week.

Drink Plenty of Clean Water Every Day

Your body is two-thirds water. Think of that water as a crystal clear mountain lake. Now imagine that lake becoming stagnant because the streams that bring water into and out of it stop flowing. A stagnant lake becomes clouded and overgrown with algae. Now, imagine a campground being built next to the lake, bringing with it trash and sewage. More and more toxins come in, and there is no moving fresh water to flush them away. Eventually, the lake becomes uninhabitable to the life forms that once thrived there.

This is what happens in your body when you eat lots of processed foods high in sugar and fat, and when you don't drink enough water. If you don't constantly flush toxins from the water that makes up much of your body, they build up and can cause chronic disease. Even if you eat a whole-foods diet, you're still exposed to plenty of environmental toxins.

Drinking six to eight 8-ounce glasses of *pure* water a day—not coffee, not juice, not milk, but water—is one of the simplest things you can do to improve your health. (Tap water simply isn't safe to drink. Depending on where you live and where your water comes from, the types of toxins that flow from your tap will vary. Heavy metals, benzene, chlorine, and carcinogenic agricultural chemicals are typical findings in tap water. Bottled water is expensive, and its quality isn't always assured. Anyone serious about improving his or her health should buy a water-filtration system.)

Eat Less, Enjoy Life More

Research is revealing that eating too much food for years on end not only can make us overweight, but can also make us age prematurely. Studies of animals and humans with low caloric intakes show that they are far less likely to fall prey to heart disease, cancer, and other chronic diseases, such as arthritis. They live longer and have more energy. The research also shows that caloric intake over a whole lifetime is the important thing. Whether we periodically overindulge and make up for it with a fast or simply refrain from overeating in general, we can still enjoy the benefits of longer life and less chronic disease. Eating less also reduces excess weight, which relieves stress on arthritic joints.

GUARD AGAINST LEAKY GUT

In Chapter 3, you read about how NSAIDs can create tiny holes in the wall of the small intestines. These holes allow toxins and incompletely digested bits of food to pass into the bloodstream. These are substances that probably would never get through the tightly knit, highly selective boundary of an intact intestinal wall. Once toxins and undigested food particles get into the circulation, immune cells tag them as foreign and attack them. From that point, the body may consider perfectly harmless foods as enemies to be attacked.

If toxins become lodged in joint tissues, they could conceivably start an autoimmune response in that joint. This is one theory about how rheumatoid arthritis gets started. A more generalized immune response throughout the body can mean increased sensitivity to toxins in general. It's thought that this could be a contributing factor in severe environmental allergies and asthma.

Food Allergies

When the body becomes sensitized to a particular food, the intestinal immune system begins to react to it strongly. The inflammation that results can eat small holes into the intestinal wall. Wheat, gluten, yeast, dairy products, eggs, soy, beef, peanuts, and nightshade vegetables (tomatoes, potatoes, red and green peppers, eggplant, tobacco, coffee, and corn) are common food allergens.

You may have noticed that the foods most likely to cause allergies are those that many people eat every day, or even at every meal. Ironically, it's usually the foods you love the most and feel you couldn't live without that you become allergic to. Most food allergens happen also to be found in a great many processed foods. The allergic reaction creates a mild stimulant effect, and so we may feel addicted to these foods.

Immediate food allergies cause sneezing, hives, runny nose, wheezing, watery, itchy eyes, or *anaphylaxis* (a swelling of the airways that can be life threatening if not treated immediately). Immediate food allergies, usually to strawberries, peanuts, beans, seafood, or dairy, generally occur in children and are often outgrown.

Delayed food allergies, on the other hand, affect adults and cause more subtle symptoms. It's difficult to connect them to the offending food, because the symptoms may take some time to develop. For this reason, they are referred to as *delayed* food allergies.

Fatigue, hay fever, or other environmental allergies (to animal hair or mildew, for example), indigestion, dry skin, dull hair, rashes, and other health problems that can't be attributed to anything else are often the result of delayed food allergy. Although it may not cause you to feel desperately ill, food allergy means never quite feeling your best, and certainly can compromise your quality of life.

The Elimination Diet

Most conventional medical doctors aren't yet aware of leaky gut and delayed food allergies or how to treat them. However, there is plentiful evidence that when people with chronic illnesses, including arthritis, take steps to identify food allergens and eliminate them, they experience significant improvements in their health. Fortunately, identifying your food allergies is something you can do on your own with what's known as an *elimination diet*. If you have rheumatoid arthritis, the elimination diet is an especially important step for you to take on the path to healing.

Identifying and eliminating food allergens with an elimination diet takes discipline, attention to detail, and a willingness to deprive yourself of the pleasure of eating the foods you love, at least temporarily. It isn't nearly as easy as taking pills to suppress symptoms. Going on the elimination diet will, however, benefit your health immeasurably, teach you to appreciate new foods, and guide you to lifelong dietary changes that will encourage your joints to heal.

Start out by continuing to eat your normal diet. Write down everything you eat or drink for a period of ten days. If you eat a lot of processed foods, try to keep good records of the ingredients they contain. For example, if you have a packaged cinnamon roll for breakfast every day, it probably contains wheat flour, milk, and eggs—all common food allergens.

After a week's time, sit down with your diet record and make a few categories: one for foods you eat at every meal; one for foods you eat every day; and one for foods you eat five or more times a week. Now you know which foods you ought to eliminate. Start out by eliminating the foods that appear in all three categories. If you're eliminating wheat, cut out all gluten-containing grains, including wheat, barley, spelt, kamut, and oats. Wheat is one of the hardest things to eliminate, since it's hidden in so many products, such as soups and even condiments. (Flours made from rice, corn, and potatoes do not contain gluten.)

You may find it difficult to figure out what to eat during the weeks of the elimination diet. Focus on fresh, in-season, organic vegetables and fruit, all the varieties of brown rice (a grain that is usually the staple of a nonallergenic diet), deep-water fish such as salmon, cod, and mackerel, and small servings of free-range chicken. Meat is also okay, although some people are sensitive to beef. Carefully read the labels of any

A Note about the Nightshade Family

One popular theory about diet and arthritis involves allergy to the *nightshade vegetables*. This family of vegetables includes eggplant, corn, coffee beans, tomatoes, potatoes, red and green peppers, tobacco, and cayenne pepper. Eliminating these foods has helped people with osteoarthritis and rheumatoid arthritis. It's thought that the *solanum alkaloids* in these foods can cause osteoarthritic or inflammatory changes in the joints of people who are sensitive to them. If you eat any of these foods frequently, make sure to include the entire family on your list of foods to eliminate.

processed foods you choose. Go to your health food store and have a clerk help you stock up on quick, convenient staples such as rice noodles and organic soups. There are many more choices than ever before for people on restricted diets.

Eat slowly and deliberately. Take small bites, chew your food completely, and enjoy its tastes and textures. Don't fall into the pattern of eating the same foods day after day; rotate your new staple foods. Of course, you should drink plenty of water throughout the day. Keep a written record of what you eat. Also write down how you are feeling and whether you notice my changes in your symptoms.

After two weeks, it's time for the food challenges, where you reintroduce the foods you have eliminated, one at a time. Don't challenge more than one food in a twenty-four-hour period. Have only the food you're testing at a single meal. If you are trying to discern whether you have an allergy to wheat, have a bowl of plain cream of wheat cereal or cooked wheat berries. If it's dairy you suspect, have a glass of organic milk, and so on.

Because your system has been emptied during the elimination period of all food allergens, your reaction to the reintroduced allergen will be more pronounced. Some of the more common symptoms people experience when reintroducing foods on an elimination diet are fatigue, headache, uneven or unusually fast heartbeat, muscle or joint aches, stomach cramps, bloating, diarrhea, gas, constipation, chills, sweats, and rashes. These can occur almost immediately or in a matter of hours. If you have these or other unusual symptoms when you reintroduce a food, there's a good chance you're allergic to it.

You may find that your health improves dramatically once you cut processed foods with artificial flavorings and colorings out of your diet. If this is what you find, and none of the food challenges yields results, you may have sensitivities not to the foods themselves but to the additives, preservatives, and dyes. Many people are allergic to yellow and red dyes in particular. Avoiding these chemicals permanently is the best solution.

Once you've figured out what foods set you off, avoid them completely for two months. Chances are, you'll feel much better than you did before going on the limited diet. After two months, test the foods again. If you have a reaction again, go off the foods for six months before trying again. This will allow your body to lose its sensitivity, and eventually you should be able to enjoy the foods you eliminated once in a while—but not every day.

Supplements to Relieve Leaky Gut

If your food allergies have caused leaky gut, there are some supplements you can use to help your intestines heal. Glutamine, an amino acid, is the intestinal wall's favorite fuel; taking 500 mg three times a day between meals will give the gut cells the energy they need to reestablish a healthy lining. Supplements to control inflammation in the intestines are also a good idea during an elimination diet. You'll find out more about anti-inflammatory supplements and natural remedies in Chapters 7 and 8. Vitamin B_5 (pantothenic acid) is needed by the intestinal wall to build healthy cells. Take 500 mg twice a day during the first two weeks of your elimination diet.

Yeast Overgrowth

Yeast (*Candida albicans*) grows in the small and large intestines. It normally coexists peacefully with the other organisms there. If probiotic bacteria populations drop, yeast can become overgrown. *Candidiasis* damages the delicate lining of the intestines, contributing to leaky gut and allowing bacteria to pass into the circulation. Yeasts pump out toxic byproducts that can seep through the intestinal walls, and the immune system is forced to constantly work overtime to get rid of toxins released by the yeast.

Chronic, low-grade candida overgrowth is another disorder that has been almost completely overlooked by conventional medicine. Yet, it's well-established that yeast overgrowth is often found in people with arthritis, autoimmune diseases, constipation, irritable bowel syndrome, heartburn, gas, menstrual problems, out-of-control allergies, food allergies, sugar cravings, sinusitis, rashes, fingernail or toenail fungus, and inflammation of the urinary tract. If you have health problems like these that you can't find any explanation for, you may have yeast overgrowth.

What kills off probiotic bacteria and allows yeast to run rampant? One major culprit is the standard American diet. A diet high in refined carbohydrates (yeast's favorite food) and low in fiber encourages yeast overgrowth and stifles the growth of probiotics. Antibiotics also kill off good bacteria, allowing yeast to flourish, and birth control pills set up hormonal imbalances that allow yeast to flourish. Oral steroid drugs also have this effect. If you have used any of these drugs for any length of time, there's a greater probability of your having yeast overgrowth.

Just as many people dramatically improve their health with elimination diets, many others do so by taking steps to get yeast overgrowth under control. (In fact, many of those who have leaky gut also have yeast overgrowth.) Doing so can only help; it involves changing your diet and taking a few natural supplements. Relief of pain and inflammation in rheumatoid arthritis and osteoarthritis are among the benefits of restoring order to the intestinal ecosystem.

The approach here is simple: cut way down on refined grains and sugar, use a probiotic supplement with *fructooligosaccharides* (carbohydrate molecules that are good nutrition for friendly bacteria), and wean yourself off antibiotics, birth control pills, and oral steroid drugs. You can find a good refrigerated probiotic supplement in your health food store. Take it according to the directions on the container. Also eat foods fortified with *lactobacillus* and *bifidus* bacteria, such as live-culture yogurt, kefir, unpasteurized miso, and sauerkraut. Bananas are an excellent source of fructooligosaccharides.

Fasting for Rheumatoid Arthritis

Fasting can have remarkable curative effects on rheumatoid arthritis. Abstaining from food and drink (except for water) may seem like a drastic approach to controlling inflammation, but it works. The elimination diet outlined above also will work to curb the progression of an rheumatoid arthritis flare-up, but total fasting will yield more dramatic results more quickly.

Fasting has been a part of religious observances throughout history and has been used to treat disease almost as long. Ancient Greek medical tests, upon which modem medicine is based in many ways, prescribe fasting for the treatment of a variety of diseases. Not eating for three to seven days may sound impossible and risky, but most humans can go without food for up to forty days without any significant ill effects.

Any fast lasting more than three days should be supervised by a physician. This is especially true of those who are using medications. Drugs commonly used for rheumatoid arthritis, including NSAIDs and corticosteroid drugs, are likely to cause serious kidney damage if taken during a fast. If you are using medications, you will need to work with a physician to wean yourself off of the drugs to be sure you can fast safely. Some people cannot fast safely at all and are better off simply shifting to an organic whole-foods diet. During the course of a fast, the physician will monitor your blood pressure and blood levels of electrolytes (minerals). If either of these tests show dangerous changes, your doctor will help you terminate the fast properly.

When you undergo a fast, your body has a rare opportunity to reestablish balance, without the stress of digesting and assimilating food three or more times a day. In his book, *Fasting—and Eating—for Health* (St. Martin's Griffin, 1998), Joel Fuhrman, M.D., says it succinctly: "Therapeutic fasting . . . works because the body has within it the capacity to heal once the obstacles to healing are removed."

It's very important to properly prepare for and break a fast. Two weeks on a whole-foods diet, tapering down to only vegetables, fruit, and rice, is the best way to ease into a fast with the least trauma to the body. At the end of a long fast, you'll need to break it carefully, starting out with small meals of easy-to-digest vegetables and fruits, and cooked whole grains, and adding fats, seeds, and protein foods in gradually, increasing amounts two to three days after the fast has ended.

After the second or third day of a fast, feelings of hunger dissipate, and a shift takes place—the body's energy needs are filled by stored fuel. Internal changes are made to preserve muscle tissue and provide energy from stored fat. This mode is also a cleansing mode. Detoxification processes, relieved of the constant work of processing meal after meal throughout the day, have a chance to clear out stored wastes from body tissues. Liver function and immune system function are both improved during a fast.

Judicious use of enemas is helpful in the cleansing process, as are dry-brushing the skin before showering and alternating hot and cool water in the shower. While fasting, get as much rest as you can, avoid stress, and take plenty of naps.

If a long fast seems too daunting or is impossible for you because of medications or other factors, there are less drastic approaches you can take. Periodic one-day water fasts are safe for nearly everyone, with the exception of insulin-dependent diabetics. Those who don't wish to go without food can try a one-day to one-week cleansing diet consisting only of fresh organic vegetables, fruit, water, and tea. While extended fasts are more potent medicine than these other approaches, you'll still gain considerable benefit. Another plus for those who wish to try the shorter fasts or cleansing diets: you won't need a doctor's supervision.

An excellent resource on fasting and elimination diets is the book *Optimal Wellness* by Ralph Golan, M.D. (Wellspring/Ballantine, 1995).

Side Effects of Fasting

It isn't uncommon for people who are fasting to experience nausea, headaches, strange body odors, itching, rashes, fatigue, congestion, aches and pains, dark urine, foul-smelling bowel movements, and other unpleasant symptoms. As the body burns up stores of fat, toxins are set loose in the circulation before they are detoxified or excreted, and they can't be eliminated fast enough. They can rise to high enough levels in the body that you'll feel worse before you feel better. The more symptoms you experience, the more toxicity you've been carrying around in your body, and knowing that you're getting it out of your system may be some small consolation.

CHAPTER 5

Nutritional Supplements for Pain-Free Joints

*T*he practice of treating disease with vitamin and mineral supplements, known as *orthomolecular medicine,* began in earnest with two-time Nobel laureate Linus Pauling's groundbreaking research on vitamin C in the late 1960s and 1970s. He found vitamin C to be a valuable treatment for the common cold, and also found that high doses of the vitamin dramatically prolonged the lives of terminal cancer patients. Since Dr. Pauling proposed the use of high doses of vitamins and minerals for the prevention and treatment of disease, an entire community of researchers and health practitioners has followed suit.

Today, naturopaths and complementary medicine physicians commonly prescribe supplemental nutrients to treat illness. This is not because they work as "magic bullets," but because they support and strengthen the body in ways that naturally bring us back to health. Due to the successes achieved with the orthomolecular approach, research efforts in this area have expanded. The science behind it has led to better acceptance of orthomolecular therapies by conventional medicine and literally thousands of scientific studies show the benefits of these types of approaches.

If you are committed to enjoying optimal health and relief from symptoms of arthritis, be prepared to add nutritional supplements to your whole-foods diet. Vitamin and mineral supplements ensure that your body never lacks the nutrients it needs to perform all of its functions smoothly. A typical argument against supplements is that a healthy diet can supply all we need of these nutrients. This may be true of those who live in ideal conditions, with clean air and water, who eat a diet composed only of whole, fresh, organic foods grown in mineral-rich soil, and who don't suffer from much stress. The rest of us must contend with foods that have been grown in depleted soil and that have lost many of their nutrients from sitting on shelves and being cooked or processed. Pollution, toxic chemicals, and unprecedented levels of stress increase our need for certain nutrients. Nutritional supplements give us the support we need to stay healthy in an environment that is anything but healthful.

When you make the decision to use nutritional supplements to treat a disease such as arthritis, your expectations may need a little adjustment. After all, we've been led to believe that every disease treatment should work fast to eliminate uncomfortable symptoms. When you use nutrients, the beneficial effects appear gradually and with more subtlety as your body's healing systems are gently stimulated and supported. It can take months to notice a difference, even when you are religiously following your supplement plan. Sometimes, results are quick and dramatic. If they aren't, remember—it took you years to create this disease, so give your body some time to heal.

ANTIOXIDANTS

Vitamin C

Research has shown that elderly people with cartilage disorders are usually deficient in vitamin C. This vitamin is needed to make collagen, the basic building block of all connective tissues. In studies on both animals and humans, high intakes of vitamin C reduced joint inflammation, decreased the rate of cartilage deterioration, and reduced the likelihood of joint pain. This vitamin appears also to stimulate the growth of cartilage and the production of anti-inflammatory prostaglandins.

Vitamin C is acidic, and high doses can cause stomach upset or diarrhea. If this is a concern for you, use a buffered version, such as calcium ascorbate or magnesium ascorbate. The cheapest way to buy vitamin C is as a powder, which you can stir into juice. Chewable vitamin C can damage tooth enamel. Also, consult your doctor about using high doses (over 500 mg per day) of vitamin C if you are taking diabetes medications. Too

Antioxidants and Free Radicals

As you've learned, free radicals are submicroscopic particles that can cause damage to cells. They are formed in the process of normal metabolism as cells transform protein, carbohydrate, and fats into energy. They are also formed for specific jobs; for example, the immune system creates free radicals to help with the job of warding off infectious disease. Free radicals are plentifully created during the process of inflammation, and they are thought to play a significant role in both rheumatoid and osteoarthritis (see Chapter 2).

If antioxidants are readily available in the body, free radicals shouldn't build up enough to do any appreciable damage. Once the antioxidant has quenched a free radical, it becomes a free radical itself and needs to be replenished by another antioxidant. Different antioxidants have different specialties. Some target the free radicals formed when fats are oxidized; others protect the liver from oxidation; others are especially good at replenishing other antioxidants. That's why it's so important to get a full spectrum of antioxidant nutrients—vitamins C, E, and beta-carotene especially—in adequate amounts.

The foods richest in antioxidant nutrients are vegetables and fruits. Most antioxidant supplements are derived from these foods. Humans also make endogenous antioxidants, including glutathione and superoxide dismutase (SOD). These antioxidants aren't found in foods, but nutrients found in foods and supplements—including zinc, copper, and sulfur—are needed to make the endogenous antioxidants.

much vitamin C can counteract the effects of the medicine. Use from 1,000–3,000 mg a day in divided doses.

Quercetin

This antioxidant is part of a family of plant compounds called *bioflavonoids*. Bioflavonoids were once thought to simply increase the absorption of vitamin C. Now we know that the bioflavonoid nutrients are powerful antioxidants on their own and have great value in the treatment and prevention of inflammatory diseases. Quercetin, for example, suppresses inflammation in joints affected by rheumatoid arthritis, essentially by breaking the chain of events that cause the inflammatory process to balloon out of control. Those with osteoarthritis will benefit from quercetin's potency as an antioxidant.

Products containing both quercetin and bromelain (a protein-digesting enzyme) are available. Try one that gives you 500 mg each of bromelain and quercetin. Use it twice a day.

Oligomeric Proanthocyanidins (OPCs)

Cranberries, bilberries, blueberries, blackberries, cherries, and red and purple grapes are examples of fruits that are rich in these plant pigments. Grape-seed extract also contains them. OPC supplements are also made from French maritime pine-tree bark, sold under the brand name Pycnogenol. The OPCs are incredibly powerful antioxidants. They readily donate elections to oxidized vitamin C, reactivating it. On their own, they have been shown to have eighteen times the effectiveness of vitamin C and fifty times the effectiveness of vitamin E at neutralizing free radicals.

In rheumatoid arthritis and osteoarthritis, newly formed collagen tends to be abnormally stiff and prone to injury with too many cross-linkages. Research has shown that OPCs promote the normal cross-linking of collagen.

The process of inflammation causes enzymes called *collagenases* to form. As the name implies, collagenases digest collagen. In healthy joints, collagenases perform a valuable function, clearing away old, damaged collagen to make room for new. In arthritic joints, collagenases appear to get carried away, digesting more than the body can replace. OPCs guard collagen from excessive collagenase activity.

Grape-seed extract is an excellent, inexpensive source of OPCs. Try taking 200 mg a day for two weeks, then a maintenance dose of 25 to 50 mg a day. Eat ripe red or purple grapes, blueberries, and cherries (organic, please!), and enjoy a glass of red wine or purple grape juice now and then. Both are rich sources of OPCs.

Vitamin E

Studies have shown that vitamin E has painkilling effects comparable to NSAIDs. Vitamin E is also the body's primary fat-soluble antioxidant.

This means that it protects cell membranes (which are composed of fats) and the fats in the blood, such as cholesterol and triglycerides, from oxidation. The synovial membrane, which is the starting place of rheumatoid arthritis inflammation, is also made up of fats, and supplying enough vitamin E is thought to protect the synovium from free-radical damage during inflammation. Early studies, performed in the 1960s, showed the potential of vitamin E to ease osteoarthritis symptoms.

Be aware that vitamin E is a blood thinner, and caution should be used if you are planning to have surgery—especially if you also happen to be taking blood-thinning medications or aspirin. If you are using either of these medications, or if you have a deficiency in the blood-clotting vitamin K, consult your healthcare provider before taking supplemental vitamin E. Anyone with an overactive thyroid (Graves' disease), high blood pressure, diabetes, or rheumatic heart disease should build up their vitamin E dose slowly, starting with 50 to 100 IU and adding 100 IU each month until 400–800 IU are taken daily.

Take 400–800 IU of natural vitamin E, also called d-alpha tocopherol. (Synthetic is dl-alpha tocopherol; please don't use it.) Vitamin E is recommended for every adult. For anti-inflammatory effects, up to 1,200 IU a day have been used, but you should not use more than 800 IU a day without a doctor's guidance.

Vitamin A and the Carotenes

Vitamin A, found in fish, butter, milk, and organ meats, is available in supplement form. Vitamin A stimulates the immune system and can be a powerful ally in fending off infections and healing infections and wounds. High doses of vitamin A—more than 50,000 IU per day for more than a week or two—can lead to toxicity. Women who are pregnant or may become pregnant should not use more than 15,000 IU of vitamin A per day. However, doses of 10,000–15,000 IU a day are quite safe and are an important part of every adult and child vitamin regimen.

Low levels of vitamin A and beta-carotene, a nutritional precursor of vitamin A, increase risk of autoimmune diseases in general. In most people, beta-carotene can be turned into vitamin A once it's in the body, but it also has many functions of its own.

Beta-carotene is one of about 600 carotenes. The carotenes are plant pigments, found plentifully in bright yellow and orange vegetables and fruits, some of which can be transformed into vitamin A in the body. The antioxidant activity of the carotenes is much greater than that of vitamin A. Beta-carotene is the best known of the carotenes and is most easily transformed to vitamin A, but there are at least thirty different carotenes that can undergo the conversion.

A mixed carotenoid supplement, including beta-carotene, lycopene, alpha-carotene, gamma-carotene, lutein, and zeaxanthin, will lend antioxidant support to arthritic joints. Eating plenty of brightly colored vegetables and fruits will also increase your carotene intake.

HEALTHY FATS

Omega-3 Fats (Eicosapentaenoic Acids; EPAs)

You've already learned about the importance of getting plenty of EPAs in your diet. EPAs are the raw material from which anti-inflammatory eicosanoids are built. Low levels of EPAs have been found in the bodies of people with inflammatory diseases and studies have shown that supplemental EPAs can help decrease autoimmune inflammation. Some of the subjects in the studies that back this therapy up were able to decrease their NSAID dosages with fish oil supplementation.

Most EPA supplements are derived from fish oils. The problem with fish oil supplements is that they go rancid—in other words, they oxidize—quite easily. Taking a rancid fish oil supplement is equivalent to swallowing a mouthful of free radicals, in which case the fish oil will do more harm than good. Even if you are able to protect it from heat and light and keep it in the refrigerator, the fish oil may have already become partly oxidized during processing. Another drawback to supplementation is that the recommended dose for treating rheumatoid arthritis symptoms is quite high—3 to 7 grams of fish oil a day (or 1.8 grams of EPA) for three to twelve months—and this can get expensive and be very unpleasant if it burps back up.

The best way to get your EPAs is by eating deepwater fish, and by cutting down on sources of fat that are transformed into pro-inflammatory eicosanoids—saturated fats from red meats and dairy products, hydrogenated fats, and vegetable oils. Your goal is to raise levels of omega-3s and decrease levels of pro-inflammatory fats. Whether you have osteoarthritis or rheumatoid arthritis, improving your balance of healthy fats in this way will improve your overall health.

For some people with rheumatoid arthritis, EPA supplementation with fish oil may be worth a try, because much higher doses of EPA can be concentrated in a capsule than can be obtained through the diet. Just be sure that it's well preserved. Break open a capsule and smell it—if it smells rancid (versus just fishy), find another brand.

Flaxseed Oil

For raising omega-3 levels, some health experts recommend supplemental flaxseed oil over fish oil. Flax oil contains another type of omega-3 fatty acid, alpha-linolenic acid (ALA). In order to serve as raw material for the anti-inflammatory eicosanoids, ALA must be converted to EPA in the body. Flax oil supplementation doesn't raise blood levels of EPA as much as fish oil does. However, if you decrease your intake of polyunsaturated vegetable oils—that means safflower, sunflower, and corn oils, used in many high-fat processed foods—flax is move effective at raising the level of EPA. But a problem with flaxseed oil is that it is one of the most unstable oils in existence—so much so that by the time you get it home from the store, it's probably rancid.

One good way to include flax in your anti-inflammatory regimen is to buy whole flaxseeds. Within the seed are antioxidant substances that protect the fats from becoming oxidized. You can grind them into a fine meal in a coffee grinder and sprinkle them onto salads, cereals, and soups. Keep the seeds in the refrigerator. Buy only small amounts at a time, and grind them only as needed. This is an excellent way to add nutritious, fiber-rich whole seeds to your diet.

It is important that you do not use too much flax oil, or it could have the opposite effect you intended, increasing the free-radical load in the body. Remember, Mother Nature has seen fit to package these types of oils in very small amounts, mainly in vegetables, nuts, seeds, and whole grains. In tiny amounts they're much needed, but in high amounts they can be destructive. The imbalance of fats and oils found in North American culture is caused more by an excess of saturated fats and hydrogenated oils, and virtually none of the other types of oils. The idea is to strive for balance. If you cut out hydrogenated oils altogether and eat a moderate amount of saturated fat and monounsaturated oils and plenty of fresh vegetables, nuts, seeds, whole grains, and fish, your fatty acid balance should be fine.

Omega-6 Fats

These fats are rich in gamma-linolenic acid, or GLA. They are found in safflower, sunflower, and soybean oils, and are also sold as supplements made from evening primrose, black currant, or borage oils. Omega-6 fats can be transformed into either "good" or "bad" eicosanoids, depending on the presence of certain enzymes. Because it isn't known exactly how to ensure that omega-6 fats go into making good eicosanoids, there is some controversy around its use in the treatment of rheumatoid arthritis.

Studies on rheumatoid arthritis patients lasting up to one year have shown significant improvements in pain, swelling, morning stiffness, and the number of tender and swollen joints with very high supplemental doses of GLA. Results of GLA studies haven't been consistent, however, and it has been shown that long-term supplementation of omega-6 oils can lead to decreases in levels of EPA (the fats that turn into "good" eicosanoids) and increases in levels of arachidonic acid (the fats that turn into "bad" eicosanoids). Most people get plenty of omega-6 oils in the form of vegetable oils and don't need additional GLA.

ENZYMES

Supplementation of dietary enzymes, which are a part of all fresh plant foods, is often beneficial to people with rheumatoid arthritis. They are thought to work by slowing down inflammatory reactions themselves, and by activating immune cells that do the same. There is some scientific evidence in favor of dietary enzyme therapy for rheumatoid arthritis. Pain from muscle injuries, which usually involves inflammation, has also been shown to respond well to bromelain.

Many people find that 100 to 500 mg of bromelain (a protein-digesting enzyme derived from pineapple) three times a day between meals improves their mobility and decreases their joint swelling. Protein-digesting enzymes seem to work best. Pancreatin, papain, and trypsin are other protein-digesting enzymes you might want to try. If you find that the enzymes make you nauseated, try taking them with meals instead of between meals. Once you stop taking it, symptoms that were relieved by the enzyme supplement are likely to return—so if it works for you, keep using it. Supplements that contain 500 mg of bromelain and 500 mg of quercetin per dose are ideal.

OTHER NUTRITIONAL SUPPLEMENTS

Vitamin D

This vitamin is needed for proper absorption of calcium and the building of healthy bones and cartilage. Damage to bones and cartilage is an end result of both rheumatoid arthritis and osteoarthritis, and low vitamin D levels have been found in people with arthritic diseases. In some research circles, it's thought that a defective gene may alter the action of vitamin D in the body, increasing the likelihood that those with the defect will end up with arthritis. Problems with vitamin D activity affect the cells that make cartilage and bone in joints affected by both types of arthritis, increasing the rate at which bone is broken down there. Vitamin D supplementation is an important preventative measure against osteoporosis.

If you are using vitamin D supplements derived from fish oil, check to see how much vitamin D they contain—you don't want to get too much. Vitamin D is a fat-soluble vitamin and can build up in the body to toxic levels. (Excess water-soluble vitamins are simply flushed away in the urine, while fat-soluble vitamins are stored away.)

Most adults under fifty should supplement with 400 IU a day, and those over fifty should take 800 IU a day. If you get a daily dose of sunshine you can probably get by on 400 IU.

Niacin

The B vitamin niacin has been used in orthomolecular medicine to relieve rheumatoid arthritis and osteoarthritis symptoms since the 1950s. Very few clinical studies have been done to support its use for this purpose, but those that have been done have shown promising results. In one study, with 500 mg of niacin six times per day, joint mobility improved, and pain and the need for NSAIDs decreased. If you want to try high-dose niacin, start out by taking 50 mg of no-flush niacin (inositol hexaniacinate) three times a day with meals. You can gradually increase the dose up to 100 mg three times a day, but do so gradually, over the span of a month. Some people can tolerate as much as 300 mg daily, but this should only be taken under the supervision of a healthcare professional. Be sure to let your doctor know you are using niacin, especially if you have gout, stomach ulcers, liver disease, glaucoma, or severe diabetes.

Methylsulfonylsufate (MSM)

In addition to ginger, which you'll read read about in the next chapter, MSM is one of the most exciting nutritional supplements available for the treatment of rheumatoid and osteoarthritis symptoms. The potential uses of MSM are many: it relieves pain and inflammation; improves blood flow by dilating blood vessels; reduces formation of scar tissue; improves health of skin, hair, and nails; helps normalize the immune system; reduces muscle spasms; and even has some anti-parasite activity.

Ever soaked in a hot sulfur spring? If you have, you know how soothing it can be. For centuries, people have sought sulfur springs because of their healing effect on arthritic diseases, skin conditions, and even digestive disorders. MSM contains organic sulfur—the form in which the mineral sulfur occurs in living cells.

Early in the history of the therapeutic use of sulfur, another form, called DMSO, was used to treat painful joints and inflammatory diseases with notable success. The problem with DMSO was its side effects, which included a distinct garlicky odor, rash, nasal congestion, breathlessness, and allergic reactions. These side effects were bad enough to cause scientists to lose interest in researching DMSO as an arthritis remedy—that is, until the recent discovery that MSM was the main healing ingredient and could be isolated and used without these side effects.

MSM is thought to work against arthritis pain and inflammation by several different mechanisms:

- MSM donates sulfur molecules for the manufacture of collagen. Without adequate sulfur, the body can't repair the damage that happens naturally with daily wear and tear, or the accelerated damage seen in arthritis. As with many of the nutrients discussed in this chapter, sulfur levels tend to be low in people with arthritis.

- Sulfur is also a component of glutathione, the most important antioxidant made in the body. Low levels of glutathione mean decreased ability to quench free radicals that contribute to joint damage.

- It reduces muscle spasm around arthritic joints. Muscle spasm occurs in damaged joints as they try to protect themselves from further damage, and these knots can contribute a great deal to joint pain.

- MSM relieves inflammation. It is thought to have this effect due to a sensitizing effect, making the body more sensitive to its own anti-inflammatory hormones—particularly cortisol. When patients use sulfur derivatives such as DMSO and MSM, their need for cortisone drugs (synthetic pharmaceutical versions of cortisol) drops. In uncontrolled inflammation, fibroblasts (which manufacture connective tissues) work overtime, making tissues that don't function properly. DMSO, and possibly MSM, also slow down swelling and scar tissue formation by reducing the activity of fibroblasts. Sulfur compounds are also thought to remove excess fluid from sites of inflammation.

- MSM relieves pain. No one knows exactly how, but there are a few solid theories. It's been shown to inhibit the nerve impulses that send pain messages from injured tissues to the brain. Reduction of inflammation and muscle spasm also reduces pain sensations.

MSM is available as a topical cream or gel, and in powder, capsule, and tablet forms. It's well absorbed through the skin. Some proponents advise using it topically and internally at the same time for increased effectiveness. It appears that using glucosamine sulfate and MSM at the same time also has increased healing effects on arthritis.

The recommended oral dose is 1,800 to 9,000 mg a day, divided into three doses with meals. Start with the lowest dose and work up slowly, adding 300 mg each time you increase the dose. For some people, MSM works right away, and for others it takes a few weeks. The only side effects you might encounter are mild gastrointestinal upset or diarrhea. If you tend to be constipated, MSM may be just the thing for you—one of its perks is that it relieves constipation.

CHAPTER 6

The Miracle of Ginger Extract

G inger is more than a pungent, delicious spice. It's a natural remedy that has been used for more than 5,000 years to treat digestive problems and pain. In Ayurvedic medicine, ginger is part of so many herbal formulations that it is known as *vishqabbesaj,* or "universal medicine." The root, or *rhizome,* of the ginger plant contains a sticky resin packed with over 400 different biochemicals. Scientists have isolated and tested these chemicals to discover what gives ginger its healing powers, and it turns out that several of them are natural inhibitors of the formation of "bad" pro-inflammatory eicosanoids. Ginger is a sensible, effective alternative to NSAID drugs, which tear up the gastrointestinal tract. It is a gentle pain reliever that helps people who have been in chronic pain to live active, fulfilling lives once again.

In this chapter, you will learn why ginger is the superior choice over prescription and over-the-counter medications for the treatment of arthritis (and even for migraine headaches, menstrual cramps, and other inflammatory conditions). Scientific studies supporting the research of ginger extract for relieving arthritis pain and inflammation also are presented. This is followed by a discussion of the links between ginger, a healthy gastrointestinal system, and joint health.

GINGER'S RICH TRADITION

Of all the remedies in the herbalist's medicine cabinet, ginger has the longest and most colorful history. It has graced the tables of people all over the world as a spice and has been used for centuries as a healing agent. The earliest records of ginger are over five thousand years old. Since 200 B.C. this gift of nature has been used as both a culinary herb and an herbal remedy for a wide spectrum of ills. Historians have discovered records dating back to the fourth century B.C. that list many of the medical conditions treated by ginger. As a spice, ginger is a mainstay in the traditional foods of China, Japan, and other Asian countries, and its popularity has spread through many countries throughout the world. Gingerbread men and houses, as well as ginger ale and ginger snaps, are traditional parts of folktales and seasonal celebrations.

By the ninth century A.D., ginger was imported to Europe. (It could not be cultivated there because of the climate.) For many centuries, it was used there only by the wealthy. The writings of explorers Marco Polo and Vasco da Gama mention their first experiences of this exotic spice. Nations fought over trade routes for ginger, knowing that control of this wildly popular flavoring would mean riches. The thirteenth through sixteenth centuries witnessed ginger's introduction in East Africa, Malaysia, the West Indies, and other parts of Africa.

Ginger is included in ancient Arab religious texts and folklore and is still a part of some religious rituals of that culture. In the early twentieth century, anthropologists reported that natives of Papua, New Guinea, ritually spat ginger onto the roads leading into their villages for good luck. It has also been found in centuries-old tombs of Chinese monarchy, and its aphrodisiac effects are highlighted in *The Arabian Nights*. Several works of Shakespeare and Chaucer also mention ginger.

In the 1800s, a group of 25,000 physicians, collectively known as the Eclectics, popularized the medicinal uses of ginger in the United States. *The Materia Medica, Therapeutics and Pharmacognosy* by Finley Ellingwood, M.D., included the many ways in which the Eclectics reported ginger to be of use in their medical practices.

Modern science has investigated the biochemical basis for ginger's illustrious history. It has broken this herb down to its most basic components and has discovered each component's effects, both separately and in combination with each other. The more you discover about ginger, the more you will see the benefits of this time-tested natural remedy.

ALL ABOUT GINGER

Ginger was first harvested in Southeast Asia. Its scientific name, *Zingiber officinale,* was given by the famous Swedish botanist Linnaeus. It is a member of the *Zingiberacae* family, which also includes the healing herbs turmeric and cardamom (both found in curry, an Indian spice mixture). Through several linguistic twists and turns, the name "ginger" was derived from a Sanskrit word—*sringa-vera*—which describes its hornlike shape.

A graceful perennial, ginger can grow up to four feet in height. Its dark green leaves can extend to a foot in length and about three-quarters of an inch wide. Many of the plants bud with sweet-smelling purple and yellow blossoms.

Although the edible part of ginger is often referred to as its root, botanists call it a *rhizome.* Rhizomes differ from roots in that they are able to bud and grow if split and planted. Carrots and potatoes are other examples of rhizomes. In this book, the terms "ginger" and "ginger root" are used interchangeably. Different varieties of ginger may be slightly different in shape and color, and they may vary widely in the composition of their medicinal components.

More than one hundred subspecies of ginger are grown throughout southern Asia, China, Jamaica, India, and other countries where the weather is warm and moist. Ginger, which requires healthy, rich soil, draws a great many nutrients into its rhizome as it grows. Most commercially available ginger is cultivated. It must be allowed to grow for at least six months to be useful, because it takes that long for the oils, which are believed to contain most of its medicinal components, to fully develop. Optimally, ginger should be allowed to grow and mature for nine months. At this point, it is bursting with over 400 biochemicals, many of which are valuable healing agents.

GINGER AS MEDICINE

Confucius wrote about ginger's benefits for aiding digestion, and two Chinese medical texts dating from A.D. 500 mention its medicinal uses. Western herbalists have made ginger a part of their natural pharmacies since the 1800s. Today, it continues to be an important ingredient in many Asian and Ayurvedic herbal formulations.

In our modern medical age of laboratory-produced, chemical drugs, doctors and patients alike typically want more than a long history of or anecdotal evidence for natural remedies. They want clinical studies—scientific proof—that a remedy works. Fortunately, a growing number of researchers are taking notice of ginger and are performing studies on this remarkable herb. Scientific knowledge and proof of ginger's therapeutic value is available now.

The whitish, fibrous flesh of the ginger rhizome has been analyzed exhaustively. It is made up of 12 to 50 percent carbohydrate (more mature plants contain more carbohydrate), 6 to 8 percent fat, 9 percent protein, and 2.5 percent fiber. Enzymes—most notably a protein-digesting enzyme called *zingibain*—make up between 2 and 3 percent of this edible portion of ginger. Zingibain can break down protein at an astonishing rate. One gram of zingibain can tenderize up to twenty pounds of meat. When eaten with meat, the zingibain in fresh ginger joins forces with the enzymes secreted in the stomach and small intestine, making digestion more thorough. It's no wonder that the cuisines of Asia and India include ginger in so many of their traditional meat dishes.

Ginger is rich in vitamins, minerals, and other *phytonutrients*—chemicals found in plants that support health. It is abundant in B vitamins (including niacin and thiamine), beta-carotene, and vitamin C. Minerals found in ginger include calcium, chromium, germanium, iron, magnesium, phosphorus, selenium, and zinc. The amino acids arginine, cysteine, glycine, leucine, lysine, and tyrosine; and the health-supporting phytochemicals beta-sitosterol, capsaicin, curcumin, lecithin, limonene, and quercetin also are contained in ginger.

Essential oils give ginger its taste and aroma. These oils, which vary between the different ginger subspecies and the soil in which they are grown, make up 1 to 3 percent of the average root. Possibly the most important health-supporting component of the ginger root is the sticky oil known as *oleoresin*. Oleoresins are where the magic of the ginger root lies. They contain hundreds of compounds that have a vast array of effects on the molecular machinery of the body. It's as though nature created this herb, according to precise specifications, to help maintain good health.

Ginger oleoresin's full spectrum of ingredients is lengthy, but its most fundamental constituents are the *gingerols*. Gingerols, of which there are more than twenty different types, make up approximately 33 percent of fresh ginger oleoresin. They are proving to be the most therapeutically valuable of ginger's chemical building blocks. You'll learn more about the beneficial effects of gingerols as you read on.

As scientists discover more about ginger's active ingredients, this knowledge is being used to create formulas for treating various health conditions. A number of researchers have been fascinated by ginger's positive effects on joint health. After meticulously testing the effects of each of ginger's active ingredients on joint health, one biochemist in particular, Dr. Morton Weidner, formulated an extract that is proving to be even more effective on arthritis and other inflammatory joint diseases than ginger root alone.

Scientists usually start with plant extracts and then attempt to isolate the active ingredients that have some therapeutic effect on the body. What these so-called "active" ingredients usually lack are the plant's *synergistic ingredients*—the other plant substances that help the active ingredients perform their functions. *Nutraceuticals* are natural therapeutic products that contain substances that exist in nature, but in order for them to be classified as prescription drugs, their active ingredients must be isolated in a lab. Once they have been chemically altered, they are unlike anything found in nature. This is the major difference between prescription arthritis drugs and nutraceuticals: nutraceuticals like ginger extract include synergistic ingredients necessary to optimize the health-promoting effects of the active ingredient, while prescription drugs are isolated compounds.

As previously discussed, the active ingredients of prescription drugs are often derived from plants. In order to create a "patentable" pharmaceutical, the manufacturer must somehow alter the molecules so that they are no longer completely natural. Most natural substances are not patentable, so they can't be priced competitively. Pharmaceutical companies end up changing the molecules into something the body doesn't recognize and something that isn't well-matched to the body's natural systems. This is one reason for the very high frequency of side effects seen with prescription drugs.

GINGER—NATURE'S ANTI-INFLAMMATORY

Today, ginger is a component of over fifty different herbal remedies throughout the world. It has been used for centuries to relieve joint pain, headaches, sore throats, menstrual cramps, and toothaches. But it was the work of Danish researcher Dr. K. C. Srivastava in the 1980s that provided sound scientific basis for ginger's role in easing the pain and inflammation of arthritis. His work has served as a springboard for many scientists, including biochemist Dr. Weidner (see page 85), in isolating the ginger components that help relieve arthritis symptoms.

In one study involving laboratory rats with severely arthritic paws, Dr. Srivastava found that daily doses of ginger oil and eugenol—a constituent of ginger—significantly reduced the arthritis within thirty days. In a test-tube study, he found that the ginger extract reduced *lipoxygenase* formation. (As explained in Chapter 2, lipoxygenase is the enzyme that creates "good" and "bad" leukotrienes and the COX-2 enzyme.) Another study involved fifty-six patients–twenty-eight with rheumatoid arthritis, eighteen with osteoarthritis, and ten with general muscle pain. After taking powdered ginger for a minimum of three months, all the patients experienced notable relief from their symptoms.

Inflammation, Free Radicals, and Ginger

As you know, free radicals accelerate the inflammatory process. Immune cells gathering at the site of inflammation stimulate the formation of inflammatory eicosanoids, which, in turn, cause more free radicals to form. Free radicals are destructive to joint tissues and to *hyaluronic acid*–the slippery joint-protective fluid that prevents damaging friction in the joints. Antioxidant substances from the ginger rhizome interrupt this cycle, helping to prevent free-radical formation from spinning out of control.

Dr. Morton Weidner, a biochemist who worked at the University of Copenhagen in Denmark, investigated the effects of ginger extract on the sudden increase in the formation of free radicals that occurs with inflammation. This "oxidative burst" is a major culprit in the permanent joint damage that occurs with arthritis. He found that at the recommended dose, ginger extract reduced the oxidative burst by about 25 percent.

Tumor necrosis factor-alpha (TNF-α) and interleukin-beta (IL1-ß)—a "bad" interleukin—are powerful inducers of inflammation. They also stimulate certain chemicals that break down collagen and generate pain. When a joint with arthritis is regularly stressed, it pumps out copious amounts of TNF-α. This doesn't happen in response to mechanical stress in a joint that does not have arthritis. In osteoarthritis patients, higher than normal levels of TNF-α are found in the joint fluid and membranes.

Ginger extract was found to stifle the inflammatory actions of "bad" inter-leukins and TNF-α.

When joints become inflamed and TNF-α and IL1–β are released, *chondrocytes* (cartilage-making cells) begin to make a particularly danger-ous type of free radical called *nitric oxide*. Nitric oxide, in turn, shuts down collagen synthesis, causing cartilage to die off. In test-tube studies, ginger extract dampened the free-radical fire of nitric oxide.

Ginger extract also stimulates the body's production of interleukin-4 (IL-4) and interleukin-10 (IL-10)—"good" interleukins that encourage the rebuilding of tissues destroyed by inflammation.

Dr. Weidner's Breakthrough with Ginger Extract

Dr. Weidner became interested in ginger as an arthritis remedy while working as a biochemist at the University of Copenhagen in Denmark. He realized how many people worldwide suffer from this disease, and he also knew the damaging side effects caused by the drugs normally pre-scribed for treating this condition. He saw the need for a natural product that could help control inflammation without negative side effects and committed himself to finding this remedy.

Starting his search in the medical library, he poured over scientific jour-nals to discover which plants had been researched for their joint-healing potential. His next step was to travel the world collecting samples of these plants for in-depth analysis in his laboratory. He visited Africa, India, Amer-ica, China, and Europe, tramping through jungles and climbing mountains to find his specimens. Back in Copenhagen, he analyzed the samples care-fully to learn which ones had the most beneficial effects on arthritic joints. A species of ginger found in China showed the most promise.

His quest led to the formulation of an extract called EV-EXT 77. This ginger extract works to soothe arthritis symptoms through several mech-anisms. It inhibits the formation of pro-inflammatory prostaglandins by about 20 percent, making it a natural COX-2 inhibitor. Unlike any of the drugs available for arthritis, EV-EXT 77 effectively prevents the pro-duction of pro-inflammatory leukotrienes that play a major role in the inflammatory process. Dr. Weidner's research showed that while the COX enzymes played a role in short-term joint discomfort, the lipoxy-genase enzymes (which lead to the formation of "bad" leukotrienes) are more instrumental in creating long-term joint discomfort. Because it suppresses both COX-2 and lipoxygenase, ginger extract is known as a dual inhibitor. It also acts as an antioxidant, calming the burst of free radicals formed when inflammation strikes.

This special herbal formulation also suppresses the formation of TNF-α, which in turn reduces pain, inflammation, and joint damage. It also encourages the formation of biochemicals responsible for the rebuilding of joint tissues damaged by inflammation. In some people, the extract works its magic within a month's time, and in others, it may take a little longer. Using fresh ginger root, powdered ginger, or whole ginger root supplements isn't going to have the same level of effectiveness against arthritis symptoms. There are over a hundred different species of ginger grown around the world, and each root's composition is different. A carefully standardized extract that is specially composed to work against arthritis symptoms is a much better bet.

Ginger extract typically is more expensive than powdered ginger or whole fresh ginger root. This is because it is standardized to the potency necessary for the desired effect. Standardized extracts are documented to contain a certain amount of the plant's active ingredients, so you know exactly what you're getting when you take them.

As mentioned earlier, ginger roots vary widely from species to species in their active ingredients. Processing further alters these ingredients. When you purchase a ginger powder or fresh root, or even a non-standardized extract to ease the pain of arthritis, there's no guarantee that the product will produce the beneficial effects of a pure standardized extract. But finally, due to Dr. Weidner's advancements, there is a reliable, well-researched, standardized ginger extract for treating inflammatory joint diseases. Visit www.DrEarlMindell.com for more information.

STUDIES ON GINGER EXTRACT

To date, there have been a number of pilot studies documenting the effectiveness of ginger extract for the relief of arthritis pain and inflammation.

In a three-month study, Danish scientist Dr. M. Norgard researched the effects of ginger extract on twenty-eight subjects who had suffered with chronic joint pain from seven to thirty-five years. By the end of the study, twenty-five displayed significant improvement. And none reported any side effects.

Another Danish scientist, Dr. Henning Bliddal, led a study at the Copenhagen Municipal Hospital. Fifty-six subjects with arthritis participated. Half of the participants were given the ginger extract, and the other half were given a placebo (sugar pill). Halfway through the study, the groups were switched, so that each group had a chance to take the ginger extract. (The subjects did not know what they were taking at any point during the study.) The results showed no change in the range of motion of the affected joints, but subjects experienced significant pain relief while taking the ginger extract compared to those using the placebo. No side effects were observed.

In Singapore, Dr. Leong Keng Hong compared the effects of ginger extract with a placebo in sixty-two arthritis sufferers. Those using the ginger extract found their symptoms had improved in only three weeks' time. There were no reports of any adverse effects.

A ten-week study conducted in tile United States analyzed the effects of ginger extract on 140 patients with arthritic knees. Half of the subjects were given ginger extract, while the other half were given a placebo. Those taking the ginger extract displayed significant improvement in knee pain compared to those taking the placebo. Again, there were no side effects.

GINGER FOR CHRONIC PAIN

Traditionally, ginger has been used for coping with and controlling chronic pain. It is believed to work by inhibiting COX-2 enzymes and any other substance that carries the chemical message of pain through the nervous system. Studies on laboratory animals have supported the use of ginger for the relief of pain from headaches, body aches, and even menstrual cramps.

Certain ginger phytochemicals inhibit the release of *substance P* a nervous system chemical that causes us to feel pain. They also inhibit the release of an enzyme called *thromboxane synthetase,* which is necessary for the manufacturing of a type of thromboxane that increases sensations of pain. When thromboxane synthetase is inhibited, the body releases another kind of hormone called *endorphins.* Endorphins are natural pain relievers. Pain relief from the use of ginger extract is, therefore, likely due to a combination of the inhibition of COX-2 enzymes, the inhibition of thromboxane synthetase, and the stimulation of endorphins.

GINGER FOR A HEALTHY DIGESTIVE SYSTEM

As you learned in Chapter 4, a healthy digestive tract is an integral part of a healthy body. In simple terms, this system is designed to absorb important nutrients found in foods and eliminate any waste. When this system does not work efficiently, toxins build up and organs don't function as they should.

Ginger's most common, traditional medicinal uses are for soothing upset stomachs and promoting proper digestion. Who hasn't been advised to sip a glass of ginger ale to help settle a queasy stomach? In addition to relieving nausea and vomiting, whether caused by pregnancy, surgery, motion sickness, or reactions to drug treatments such as chemotherapy, ginger also is a proven remedy for stomach ulcers and indigestion. Furthermore, it upholds the well-being of the small intestine and colon.

Certain properties of ginger encourage proper digestion, so it has long been a useful remedy in easing and preventing disorders of the gastrointestinal tract. Most commonly, ginger is used to ease nausea and vomiting, but it also is effective in treating stomach ulcers and other digestive system conditions.

So you have seen that ginger has a number of positive effects on the gastrointestinal system. What do the positive effects of ginger on the gastrointestinal system have to with arthritis? The answer lies primarily in ginger's effect on the small intestine. The lining of the small intestine is designed to be extremely selective. It absorbs only what the body needs and eliminates what it doesn't. At least, this is what occurs in a healthy small intestine.

Prescription drugs (particularly NSAIDs), food allergies, and poor diets that rely heavily on processed foods are the biggest culprits in eroding the intestinal lining. Eventually, this causes the formation of tiny leaks—a condition known as leaky gut syndrome that allows partially digested bits of food and chemical toxins to permeate the intestinal lining, where they enter the bloodstream. The immune system then springs into action and attacks these "foreign" invaders. However, when the immune system has to fight these invaders constantly, it gets tired and eventually is compromised. Leaky gut, in conjunction with food allergies, is associated with a number of autoimmune diseases, such as irritable bowel syndrome, chronic allergies, asthma, chronic fatigue, and arthritis. See Chapter 4 for more information on leaky gut and how to correct it.

More Positive Effects on Digestion

In addition to its important role in preventing ulcers and easing stomach upset, ginger extract is helpful in the proper absorption of nutrients in the small intestine. Ginger's constituents naturally are absorbed very rapidly through this intestinal lining. When it is taken along with food, the extract "carries" the food's nutrients with it as it is absorbed through the small intestine. In the same way, when ginger is taken with medicine, it "carries" the medicine's healing properties with it through the intestinal wall. This is one of the reasons ginger is added to so many different herbal remedies; it increases the absorption and potency of the other ingredients.

Ginger also helps enhance the body's production of bile, which further aids proper digestion. It also promotes proper transit time of digested matter. In the colon, ginger has soothing properties that help ease intestinal spasms that cause cramping. Finally, its antibacterial components support probiotic levels, encouraging their growth in the intestinal tract.

Ginger's Other Health-Promoting Effects

Not only is ginger effective in controlling joint pain and inflammation, it is both a preventive and a remedy for other types of pain, including migraine headaches and menstrual cramps. Phytochemicals that are found in the ginger rhizome may even prove important in the fight against cancer and heart disease.

Inflammation, Heart Disease, and Cancer

According to long-term studies involving the effects of NSAIDs on subjects with joint inflammation, the subjects also experienced very few incidents of cancer and heart disease. This caused researchers to investigate possible connections between runaway inflammation and the two most dangerous diseases in Western countries—heart disease and cancer.

Constricted blood vessels are a major factor in heart attacks, strokes, and chronic high blood pressure. In addition to constricted blood vessels, heart attacks and strokes also are linked to thickened blood, which typically results in dangerous blood clots, which, in turn, increase the likelihood of clogged blood vessels. Eicosanoid imbalance allows "bad" eicosanoids to cause blood components to stick together, resulting in clots. This means a greater risk of heart disease and stroke. And although NSAIDs have been effective in helping maintain the proper blood fluidity, their negative side effects on the gastrointestinal tract cannot be denied. This is another reason that treatment with ginger extract is so attractive. It has the same positive effects of NSAIDs without the harmful side effects.

Some constituents of the ginger root also are known to have cancer-preventive effects. This may be due partly to its antioxidant properties and partly to its balancing effects on eicosanoids. Since the 1970s, scientists have toyed with the idea of a link between cancer and inflammation. Deaths from colon cancer were decreased by half in large study groups in which the subjects took aspirin daily to prevent heart attacks. In another study of 2,045 women, frequent use of NSAIDs decreased breast cancer risk. And the more often NSAIDs were used, the lower the risk became. Inhibiting "bad" eicosanoids appears to have an effect against the development of cancer. Once again, because ginger extract has the anti-inflammatory efficacy of NSAIDs—without the side effects—it is clearly a better choice.

Rising cancer rates also are believed to be linked to our ever-increasing exposure to carcinogenic chemicals in the environment. Some of these chemicals become carcinogenic only when they react with certain enzymes in the gastrointestinal tract. Many of these enzymes are the same ones responsible for the formation of "bad" eicosanoids. When we inhibit these enzymes, we inhibit the formation of certain dangerous carcinogens.

Migraine Headache

Migraine headaches affect 6 percent of American men and 18 percent of American women. According to figures from the Centers for Disease Control, the prevalence of migraine headaches has risen more than 60 percent in the last twenty years.

Over half of all migraine sufferers have a family history of the condition, and they tend to experience these blindingly painful headaches between the ages of twenty and thirty-five. Intense nausea, vomiting, and dizziness often accompany migraines. In some cases, certain warning signs precede the onset of an attack, including tingling or

numbness in the body, disorientation, or extreme fatigue. Some people see sparks of light or auras around people just before a migraine
begins. The pain of these headaches can be intense and debilitating.

Unfortunately, causes of migraines and how to cure them are still
unknown. Some research points to an over-reactive system of blood
vessels in the brain. Arteries are not just hollow tubes through which
blood flows; they are well-muscled walls that narrow and expand in
response to stimulation from the nervous and hormonal systems.
During a migraine, the blood vessels just inside the skull constrict
strongly, reducing blood flow to a trickle. They then suddenly expand,
causing the nerves along the carotid artery (the major artery to the
brain) to compress, resulting in this type of intense headache. It
makes sense that eicosanoid imbalances could cause these blood
vessel changes. Changes in the electrical activity of the brain also
are believed to cause blood vessel constriction. Inflammation of
blood vessels in the brain also has been noted in migraine sufferers.
The release of certain neurotransmitters from one of the cranial
nerves causes inflammation, resulting in headache pain. Most likely,
migraine headaches are caused by a combination of these and, possibly, other factors.

In Ayurvedic medicine, ginger has a long history of neurological
benefits. It helps maintain proper eicosanoid balance, prevent blood
from dotting, and block the effects of substance P. In addition, ginger
eases two of the characteristic symptoms of migraine headaches—
nausea and vomiting.

Menstrual Pain

A number of factors are implicated in the painful sometimes debilitating cramps associated with menstruation. Typically, many women
turn to NSAIDs or synthetic estrogens for relief. Researcher Dr.
Joshua Backon observed that the prescription drug clonidine (Cat-
apres) has been shown to be effective in relieving menstrual cramps.
This drug inhibits thromboxane synthetase and stimulates the release
of the body's natural painkilling endorphins. As you have seen earlier,
ginger has the same inhibiting effects as clonidine on thromboxane
synthetase. The difference is that ginger is a natural remedy and
causes no side effects.

An Aid for Ulcers

For many years, excess stomach acid was believed to be the only cause of stomach and duodenal ulcers. It is true that studies have shown that those with duodenal ulcers have twice as many acid-producing cells as do those without this type of ulcer. However, those with gastric ulcers, which are located in the stomach, actually have normal or lower than normal stomach acid secretions. What scientists have discovered is that the use of NSAIDs, coffee, and tobacco are likely contributors to the formation of gastric ulcers. An estimated one-third of the cases of bleeding ulcers are specifically attributed to continuous NSAID use.

Recently, scientists at the University of Virginia discovered another cause of ulcers—a spiral-shaped bacteria called *Helicobacter pylori* (*H. pylori*). Found to be a major factor in many cases of ulcer, *H. pylori* attacks and wears away the mucus that protects the stomach and duodenal walls from digestive acids. Since antibiotics kill *H. pylori* they are generally part of the drug treatment for ulcers. Ginger extract is helpful in combating *H. pylori* in two ways. First, ginger has antibiotic properties itself, and second, it enhances the effectiveness of prescription antibiotics.

For preventing excess stomach acid in many ulcer patients, physicians commonly recommend antacids or histamine (H2) blockers. Antacids neutralize existing stomach acid, and H2 blockers, such as cimetidine (Tagamet) and ranitidine (Zantac) decrease the production of stomach acid. These drugs are among the top-selling ulcer drugs in the United States. Physicians also prescribe H2 blockers for the treatment of heartburn, and they are available over the counter. Both antacids and H2 blockers are often prescribed to those who are at risk for developing NSAID-related ulcers.

Using H2 blockers and antacids may help ease the discomfort of ulcers and heartburn, but not without a price. As you have seen, a certain amount of stomach acid is important for digestion. Decreasing this level disrupts the process. Acid-reducing drugs can result in incomplete food breakdown, compromised nutrient absorption, and decreased motility in moving food along the gastrointestinal tract. Worse, in many cases, these drugs mask the symptoms of ulcers, allowing them to progress.

Ginger extract is a safe, effective alternative to these drugs. Its components actually help to balance stomach acidity and pepsin secretion, rather than shutting them down like ulcer drugs. And most important, ginger causes no harmful side effects.

CHAPTER 7

Other Natural Remedies for Arthritis

*N*ature is rich with substances that have potent healing powers. In the age of high-tech medicine, natural remedies are often looked upon as primitive and rudimentary—definitely not a match for the designer chemicals commonly known as drugs. The truth is that Mother Nature can often be a far more effective healer than any modern science. Research is beginning to reveal exactly how time-tested natural remedies work to balance good health.

In this chapter, you'll find out more about natural remedies that can relieve osteoarthritis and rheumatoid arthritis symptoms. Some work by the same mechanisms as prescription drugs, while others have unique modes of action to repair damaged cartilage and counter inflammation.

There are many natural healing options for people with arthritis. Don't be daunted by the sheer number of them. They aren't meant to be tried all at once. Some are specific for rheumatoid arthritis, osteoarthritis, or both, so that should help you to narrow down your choices. Start minimally, with one or two natural remedies, and build up from there. Allow a few weeks for each to begin to work.

HELP FOR DAMAGED CARTILAGE

Glucosamine Sulfate (For Osteoarthritis)

Many of the supplements and natural remedies described in this book are designed to decrease inflammation, which is most often a characteristic of rheumatoid arthritis. Osteoarthritis symptoms may not respond as well to anti-inflammatory measures. Damaged cartilage, not inflammation, is the reason for osteoarthritis pain and disability. Any cure for osteoarthritis would have to give the body the means to repair cartilage.

Glucosamine sulfate does just that. This cartilage-supporting therapy for osteoarthritis is backed up by scientific studies performed in the United States and abroad. Glucosamine sulfate is significantly more effective than any placebo (sugar pill) at relieving osteoarthritis pain, stiffness, and swelling, and it is just as effective as NSAIDs at achieving these ends. It does this without any of NSAIDs' harmful effects on the digestive tract and without causing further deterioration of cartilage. Despite this evidence, many conventional physicians continue to deny its potential usefulness in the treatment of osteoarthritis.

Glucosamine sulfate is derived from animal cartilage. It belongs to a family of substances called *glycosaminoglycans* (GAGs)—sugars and proteins bound together. These GAG molecules link together to form *proteoglycans* (PGs). Proteoglycans, in turn, link to form connective tissue weaving through the grid work of collagen fibers. PGs are also needed to make the synovial fluid that lubricates and cushions joints.

In growing children, glucosamine and other GAGs (about 50 percent of GAGs in cartilage are glucosamine) are manufactured at a rapid clip. Throughout childhood and young adulthood, new GAGs are made as rapidly as they are worn out. In other words, in a young body, the turnover of connective tissue substances is rapid, and this keeps the joints springy and flexible. With aging, GAG production falls dramatically, and the deterioration of GAGs begins to surpass their renewal. Cartilage becomes less resilient and more easily worn down with wear and tear.

When researchers look at arthritic cartilage under a microscope, the proteoglycan chains appear worn, frayed, and shrunken in size compared to those seen in healthy cartilage. There is also less water stored in arthritic cartilage. Without an adequate fluid cushion, cartilage becomes less resilient and more vulnerable to the damaging effects of friction.

A shortage of glucosamine slows down production of GAGs and PGs, and the logic of glucosamine supplementation is to give the body what it needs to build these protein-sugar molecules. Since the early 1980s, many meticulously performed studies have shown that glucosamine sulfate supplements do in fact decrease pain and improve mobility.

They don't ultimately destroy more cartilage, as NSAIDs do, but make the building blocks of cartilage available so that the body can actually heal the joints.

Making a biochemical building block available to the body doesn't always mean that it goes to where it's needed and is property utilized. In the case of glucosamine sulfate, it not only goes to where it's needed, but it actually stimulates the formation of new cartilage. Glucosamine sulfate also stimulates the production of hyaluronic acid in synovial fluid, which keeps the fluid viscous and gives it its shock-absorbing quality. As if all of these therapeutic effects weren't enough to recommend it, glucosamine sulfate is also a mild anti-inflammatory.

Glucosamine sulfate is very well absorbed through the GI tract. The only adverse effects reported have been mild GI discomfort, drowsiness, skin reactions, and headache, but they are rarely severe enough to cause people to stop using it.

Anyone with osteoarthritis should give glucosamine sulfate a try. Buy a reputable brand, because there are a lot of less-than-ethical manufacturers jumping on the bandwagon and selling inferior supplements. Use 1,500 mg a day in divided doses. When used with MSM and antioxidants (see Chapter 6), it is even more effective at slowing the progress of, or even reversing, the course of osteoarthritis.

Chondroitin Sulfate (For Osteoarthritis)

Many advocates of glucosamine sulfate advise osteoarthritis patients to also use chondroitin sulfate. Chondroitin is another element of cartilage. It is made up of various glycosaminoglycans (GAGs), including glucosamine sulfate. Under a microscope, chondroitin is seen as short branches coming off of the pine-tree-like proteoglycan (PG) molecules. In cartilage, chondroitin and glucosamine have the same relationship as magnets turned the wrong way—they repel one another. This creates open spaces within the cartilage, which act like the open spaces in a sponge: when you squeeze the sponge, water is forced out, but as soon as you release your grip, the water returns. This is how cartilage maintains its springiness.

In aging cartilage, chondroitin chains become smaller, and less water is drawn in. Researchers have attempted to show that supplemental chondroitin would add to the positive effects of glucosamine sulfate on arthritic joints, and the results of their studies have been positive but not conclusive. A few studies have shown positive results with chondroitin sulfate alone, but most of them were performed with injected rather than oral chondroitin. This large molecule is not at all well absorbed in the GI tract, and is much more expensive than glucosamine sulfate. Try glucosamine sulfate alone for six to eight weeks. If it doesn't have the effects you were hoping for, try a supplement that will give you 1,500 mg of glucosamine sulfate and 1,200 mg of chondroitin sulfate a day.

HERBAL EXTRACTS FOR ARTHRITIS

Boswellin (*Boswellia Serrata;* Indian Frankincense) (For Rheumatoid Arthritis)

This 4,000-year-old Ayurvedic remedy relieves inflammation slightly better than the prescription NSAID phenylbutazone. It suppresses the production of pro-inflammatory eicosanoids and interrupts the chain of events that leads to out-of-control inflammation. The formation of inflammatory lipoxygenases is especially well controlled with boswellin. The therapeutic dose is 600 mg a day, in divided doses.

Cat's Claw or Uña de Gato (*Uncaria Tomentosa*) (For Osteoarthritis and Rheumatoid Arthritis)

Derived from the bark of a tree found in South America, cat's claw is a traditional Peruvian remedy for digestion problems and arthritis. It has antioxidant, anti-inflammatory, and immunity-modifying actions. It's especially useful for the treatment of osteoarthritis flare-ups. Keep it around and take 1 to 6 grams for a flare-up or drink one to two cups of cat's claw tea daily to help prevent symptoms.

Curcumin (*Curcuma longa*) (For Osteoarthritis and Rheumatoid Arthritis)

Turmeric is a bright yellow spice used commonly in Indian cooking. It has been known for its medicinal qualities for centuries. The active ingredient of turmeric is called *curcumin*. Curcumin is a very potent antioxidant and has significant anti-inflammatory effects, both of which make it an excellent candidate for relief of arthritis symptoms. Turmeric belongs to the same botanical family as ginger (see Chapter 6) and works against inflammation in much the same way—by blocking the formation of pro-inflammatory eicosanoids. Curcumin's antioxidant power nearly matches that of the oligomeric proanthocyanidins (OPCs), and it may even boost the effects of the body's natural anti-inflammatory hormone, cortisol. Use a supplement standardized to 90 percent curcumin and take 1,200 mg a day, or 600 mg at breakfast and dinner.

Feverfew (*Tanacetum parthbenium*) (For Rheumatoid Arthritis)

In Europe, this herb is often used to relieve moderate arthritis symptoms. Feverfew's flavonoids inhibit the production of cyclooxygenase and 5-lipoxygenase enzymes, which means that fewer pro-inflammatory prostaglandins and leukotrienes are created. If you would like to try it, find an extract standardized to 0.2 to 0.4 percent parthenolide and follow the instructions on the container.

HORMONES AND RHEUMATOID ARTHRITIS

Low levels of steroid hormones, such as DHEA, cortisol, and pregnenolone, have been strongly linked to increased risk of rheumatoid arthritis. No matter what type of arthritis you have, you can ask your doctor to measure your body levels of DHEA and cortisol to see whether you're deficient. If you find that you are, replacing them with supplemental hormones may be what you need to bring your body into a more youthful, healthy balance.

DHEA

DHEA (dehydroepiandrosterone) is a steroid hormone made primarily in the adrenal glands that has functions throughout the body. It is the most abundant hormone made by the adrenals. When we are in our twenties, DHEA levels are at their peak. After that, the amount of DHEA steadily declines. By the time we reach our eighties, we have about 10 percent of what we had in our young adult years. The risk of heart disease, diabetes, cancer, weakened immunity, and rheumatoid arthritis increases as levels of DHEA decrease.

Some researchers say that rheumatoid arthritis may be caused by low

DHEA and cortisol levels. Low levels of these hormones lower resistance to certain bacteria that normally exist in the body, allowing them to multiply and cause inflammation in the joints. Replacement of these hormones would, according to this theory, boost immunity and counter inflammation. Cortisol in small, physiologic doses can also have the effect of calming down an overactive and overreactive immune system.

Supplemental DHEA, just enough to restore youthful levels, has many positive effects: it improves memory, immunity, and energy, and brings about a remarkable improvement in well-being—both physical and mental. It has helped in the treatment of osteoporosis and rheumatoid arthritis.

Most of the research into the use of DHEA to treat disease has been done on animals. Although the results of that research have shown this hormone to be a promising therapy for rheumatoid arthritis, the most compelling evidence in favor of the use of DHEA is the consistency with which very low levels are found in people who have the disease. In one study, levels of DHEA were 86 percent lower in postmenopausal women with rheumatoid arthritis—and were especially low in the thirty-nine women who were taking synthetic steroid drugs.

DHEA is quite safe for people over forty in doses equal to what a youthful body makes. The recommended dose is 5 to 10 mg daily or every other day for women and 10 to 15 mg per day for men. One exception is men with prostate cancer or an abnormal PSA (prostate specific antigen) test, who should not use DHEA. Some women could develop side effects such as the growth of facial hair, male-pattern balding, or acne, because DHEA can be converted to the male hormone testosterone. If you are a woman and you experience any masculinizing side effects, cut your dose back to 2 to 5 mg every other day.

Natural Cortisols

Cortisol is a natural anti-inflammatory, and low levels predispose us to fatigue, inability to deal with stress, and inflammation. As you know, when synthetic versions of cortisol—the corticosteroid drugs such as prednisone and prednisolone—are used long-term to counter rheumatoid arthritis symptoms, the side effects can be devastating (see Chapter 3).

Endocrinologist William McK. Jefferies, M.D., has researched the possible uses and safety of natural cortisols for over thirty years. Natural cortisols are exactly like those made in the body. Rather than giving high doses to suppress inflammation, he advises his patients to use physiologic doses—only enough to reverse deficiency and restore hormone balance. In light of research showing cortisol levels to be low in rheumatoid arthritis patients, the use of natural cortisol makes sense. The case studies he describes in his book, *Safe Uses of Cortisol*, bear this out. People who had been suffering from rheumatoid arthritis for years gradually improved on 5 to 7.5 mg of hydrocortisone (Cortef) three to four times a day. If you have often had to use synthetic steroid drugs, you could benefit from natural cortisols. They are much gentler and safer.

Pregnenolone

This steroid hormone is the raw material from which all of the steroid hormones are made. Pregnenolone gives relief from arthritis symptoms to some of those who try it. There was quite a bit of research done on it in the 1940s, which was abandoned when the synthetic corticosteroids came on the market. In the studies, 100 mg two to three times a day was used. You might find it worth a try. It even has the bonus effect of improving memory.

OTHER PROMISING NATURAL REMEDIES FOR ARTHRITIS

Sea Cucumber

Sea vegetables like the sea cucumber have been used to treat arthritis in China for thousands of years. It isn't really a vegetable at all, but an animal belonging to the same family as sea urchins and starfish. Sea cucumber contains anti-inflammatory compounds that help balance eicosanoids, and also contains chondroitin and sugars called mucopolysaccharides—both components of cartilage. Use according to the directions on the container.

Green-Lipped Mussel (*Perna Canaliculus*)

In western Mexico and the South Pacific, extract of green-lipped mussels have been used in the treatment of both rheumatoid arthritis and osteoarthritis for centuries. In clinical trials, the anti-inflammatory compounds they contain have relieved pain, swelling, and stiffness in both types of arthritic disease. Use according to the directions on the container.

Cetyl Myristoleate (CMO)

In the 1970s, researchers uncovered an interesting characteristic of a specific strain of mice: they didn't get arthritis. They injected them with the same compounds consistently used to induce experimental arthritis in rats, to no avail. When they sought out what in the bodies of these mice might be protective against arthritis, they discovered a fatty acid called cetyl myristoleate (CMO).

CMO had been isolated before, but only in the bodies of sperm whales and beavers. When they isolated it from mice and injected it into rats, it effectively protected the rats from arthritis. Because it proved difficult to rally interest in an unpatentable, natural compound like CMO, the results of these studies sat untouched for years. Recently, CMO has made a comeback, and although no studies on humans have been published in major medical journals, the anecdotal reports of its effectiveness are convincing.

CMO is a fatty acid like the omega-3s and omega-6s, and appears to help eicosanoid balance. It is also thought to have a lubricating effect on joints, which makes it helpful for osteoarthritis that doesn't involve inflammation. The evidence is strong that CMO works best when used along with glucosamine sulfate. If you would like to add it to your arthritis regimen, take about 525 mg per day, or 175 mg three times a day. Take CMO with food.

HERBS AND OTHER NATURAL REMEDIES FOR PAIN AND ANXIETY

You'll probably want to keep some or all of these remedies in your herbal medicine cabinet. Some are especially effective at soothing pain; others are good for relaxation of tense muscles and for improving sleep quality.

Capsaicin (*Capsicum Frutescens* or *c. Annum*)

Cayenne pepper contains capsaicin, a chemical known to have healing properties against many chronic diseases. Capsaicin can also be found in many commercially available topical pain relievers. It deadens pain by depleting the nerves of substance P, the biochemical that transmits pain messages from the joints to the brain. If the pain messages don't travel to the brain, the pain isn't felt.

Hundreds of studies support the use of capsaicin creams for temporary pain relief. It must be applied daily for continued relief, and in some people it may take a few weeks to get results. Use a cream that contains 0.025 percent capsaicin—you should be able to find one on the shelves of your drugstore or natural foods store. Be careful not to get any residue in your eyes or mouth, because it will burn delicate mucous membranes. Wash your hands carefully right after use.

White Willow Bark (*Salicix Cortex*)

Salicylate drugs (primarily aspirin) were first derived from white willow bark. This herb is a milder, natural version of aspirin. A standardized extract containing 60 to 100 mg salicin per dose may help relieve mild osteoarthritis pain.

DL-phenylalanine (DLPA)

L-phenylalanine is an essential amino acid that is important for alertness, memory, and mood. D-phenylalanine is also an amino acid, with a special quality: it raises levels of endorphins. Remember, endorphins are natural painkillers made in the brain. When combined to form DLPA, the two have potent pain-relieving effects, especially against arthritis and back pain.

DLPA is transformed into the neurotransmitters dopamine, noradrenaline, and adrenaline, and these neurotransmitters are important regulators of mood, energy, and general well-being. To relieve chronic pain or depression, take 1,000–2,000 mg a day at first. If this isn't enough, you can take up to 3,000 mg a day. If you have high blood pressure, be sure to monitor it while using DLPA—it can cause it to rise. Only use DLPA for short-term relief (three weeks or less at a time). Long-term use can interfere with the body's balance of amino acids and can pose danger to liver and kidneys.

Valerian (*Valerian officinalis*)

This herb is a wonderfully gentle sleep aid and muscle relaxant. Herbalists have used it for centuries to relieve anxiety, panic attacks, and nervous tension. You can use it to help you sleep more deeply at night, or to relax tight, crimped muscles during the day. Don't exceed the recommended dose on the container, because high doses can cause paralysis and weakened heartbeat. Valerian can make some people weepy.

Melatonin

Melatonin is a hormone made in the pineal gland, a tiny organ nestled in the brain. It is the hormone that tells the body when it's time to go to sleep. When darkness falls, melatonin is pumped into the bloodstream, and we become sleepy.

The prevalence of electric lighting has our pineal glands quite confused. As long as rooms are brightly lit, melatonin secretion stays low. Aging also decreases our melatonin secretion. When melatonin is low, sleep quality is compromised. When you're dealing with pain, it can be hard enough to sleep as it is, and anyone who has ever lain awake at night in pain knows how awful it can be. The next day, you're irritable and tense, and your pain is made worse by your lack of sleep.

When it seems too hard to sleep through the night, use melatonin to help you fall asleep and stay asleep. A 1-mg sublingual tablet is all you'll need. Slip it beneath your tongue a half hour before going to bed.

CHAPTER 8

Therapies for Managing Arthritis Pain

We are a culture riddled with aches and pains. Americans take a staggering 30 billion dollars' worth of pain medication a year. More than 100 million suffer from some type of chronic or acute pain; of these, 37 million suffer from arthritis pain, 30 million have frequent headaches, and 15 million cope with cancer pain.

Those who suffer from chronic pain often become disabled, depressed, or angry, and relationships may suffer. It's no wonder so many turn to over-the-counter prescription drugs for relief. In this chapter, you'll out more about some natural, drug-free approaches to deal with pain.

THERAPIES FOR RELIEVING PAIN AND INFLAMMATION

Physical Therapy

Physical therapy is often prescribed after joint surgery, or to help arthritis patients strengthen weak, painful joints. The physical therapist (PT) will examine you and prescribe specific exercises to help you strengthen and stretch the muscles, tendons, and ligaments around affected joints. You'll be guided through the exercises at first, and once your therapy ends you can continue to do the exercises on your own. The exercises described in Chapter 9 are typical of the ones a PT would prescribe to you.

Physical therapy may also include hot and cold packs, whirlpool baths, massage, and TENS (transcutaneous electrical nerve stimulation). In TENS, electrodes are attached in specific places around the painful area. A mild electrical current is passed through the electrodes, and this deadens pain by a mechanism that isn't completely understood. The TENS unit is a small, battery-operated device that you can wear throughout the day once you've been trained in its proper use by a physical therapist.

Occupational Therapy

Occupational therapists (OTs) help people with physical problems accomplish their day-to-day activities. For someone with severe rheumatoid arthritis that might mean fitting a patient with special braces to support the joints and teaching him or her to use writing, cooking, and gardening utensils specially made for arthritic hands. Physical and occupational therapies are covered under most insurance plans.

Acupuncture

In Oriental medicine, it is believed that pain results from energy blockages and stagnation. This energy, called *chi,* can be redistributed and normalized by the insertion of very thin needles at specific points, depending on the location and nature of the pain. Sometimes the needles are only left in for a few minutes, or the acupuncturist may leave them in for an hour. Mild electrical currents may be passed into the needles.

Oriental medicine for pain may also include some other interesting practices, such as:

- *Guasha:* The acupuncturist scrapes the skin with a porcelain spoon.

- *Cupping:* First, the acupuncturist lights an alcohol-soaked gauze pad inside a small glass bottle, creating a vacuum. Then, the gauze is quickly removed, and the bottle is applied to specific areas of the skin.

- *Moxibustion:* Herbs are burned over—not on—painful areas.

Oriental medicine practitioners may also prescribe herbs to their patients that bring blood flow to where the pain is and direct the body's innate healing energy to those places that need it.

Clinical studies have shown acupuncture and other Oriental medicine practices to be effective at relieving pain when done by a skilled practitioner. There's more evidence in favor of its use in osteoarthritis, but there are other studies that support its use against rheumatoid arthritis pain. In two Chinese studies, researchers found that acupuncture toned down the out-of-control immune responses typical of rheumatoid arthritis.

To find an acupuncturist in your part of the world, call the American Association of Oriental Medicine at (866) 455-7999 or visit their website at www.aaom.org. You can also check your local yellow pages for licensed acupuncturists, who will have L.Ac. after their names.

Feldenkrais and Alexander Work: Movement Re-Education

Over our lifetimes, we develop unhealthy movement patterns and ways of carrying ourselves. Sitting hunched over a desk and over the wheel of a car for years and years can result in a chronically hunched posture, which is carried through all the body's movements. A shoulder injury can cause poor alignment even years after it has healed, because of habitual tensing of the muscles in an unconscious attempt to protect the shoulder from further damage. When the spine is out of alignment, it affects joints in the shoulders, hips, knees, ankles, and feet. Pain is often the result of the chronic muscle tension necessary to hold the body in unnatural alignment. These patterns may feel right to us, but only because they are habitual.

The teachings of Moshe Feldenkrais and F. M. Alexander address these issues. Therapists trained in these teachings will help you re-learn the most basic movements, many that you may never have given any conscious thought to: sitting in a chair, climbing a staircase, walking, going from sitting to lying down.

How does movement re-education relieve arthritis pain? When we don't pay attention to how we sit, stand, walk, and lie down, we adopt movement patterns and postures that put uneven stresses on the joints. These patterns don't change quickly, and it may take a few months before you experience real pain relief. But if your arthritis pain is being aggravated by the tensions in your present movement patterns, it's worth it to invest some time and energy in going to the root of those problems.

An Alexander teacher uses gentle contact with the hands to re-educate the body, while it is both still and in motion. The student has to pay close attention and participate. It's a wonderful, gentle way to get back in touch with your body and to learn to use it in the way it was designed to be used.

What Happens When You Hurt

Nerve endings called *noriceptors* are located in the skin and throughout the internal organs, joints, and bones. There can be as many as 1,300 of them in a square inch of skin. For every type of pain, there's a different type of noriceptor. Some pick up on pressure, some on heat, some on inflammation, and some on the sensation of being struck sharply. When tissues are injured by any of the above, the appropriate noriceptors send pain impulses along nerve cell pathways to the brain. Chemicals called neurotransmitters help to get the message where it needs to go.

Substance P, a protein present throughout the body, continually stimulates injured nerve endings and keeps pain messages going. When eicosanoids are out of balance, with pro-inflammatory versions predominating, nerve endings are more sensitive and transmit pain messages more quickly.

In the brain, pain impulses travel to a specialized area called the thalamus. The thalamus works as a sort of post office, collecting incoming messages and sorting them according to where they need to go next. It sends relevant information on to the cerebral cortex, the seat of thought. At this point, we can deal with the pain appropriately: for example, if you are touching a hot pan on the stove, the cerebral cortex evaluates the situation, sees the wisdom of removing your hand from the hot surface, and sends the appropriate signals to the muscles of the arm.

Messages are also sent to the limbic brain, the brain's emotional center. This is where our emotional response to pain comes into the picture. Pain is more than a physical sensation. Emotions have a lot to do with where our threshold for pain lies. Our own life experiences and our ability to deal with stress can either diminish or amplify our sensations of pain. If we react to pain with anger, increased tension, or fear, the pain can actually feel worse than if we adopt a more relaxed attitude toward it.

Sensations of pain can also stimulate the autonomic nervous system, the part of the nervous system responsible for controlling heartbeat, breathing rate, and blood flow. Stimulation causes pulse and breath rate to rise and directs blood flow away from the organs and into the muscles—the "fight-or-flight" response.

All of this is geared toward letting us know, in no uncertain terms, that something is amiss and needs attention. When we constantly mask pain sensations with drugs, we stifle this important messenger system. On the other hand, if we suffer from pain day in and day out, despite the fact that we have given it all the attention we can muster, we can seek out natural alternatives to ease the discomfort and the stress it can cause. Constant pain can seriously reduce the quality of life and make people difficult to live with. As you've learned—hopefully not firsthand—arthritis pain medications have serious liabilities and should be used only if nothing else does the job.

There are exceptions to this guideline. Pain medication can be a godsend to those on the mend from surgery or injury, who will only need it for a short time. People who are suffering from terminal cancer or other kinds of serious, uncontrollable pain should use all the pain medication at their disposal. Fear of becoming addicted or experiencing side effects shouldn't keep those who have such pain from getting relief. Cancer pain appears to be one of the only conditions for which Americans tend to be *undermedicated*.

Feldenkrais too, seeks to re-educate the body through a series of very simple exercises that feel good and increase awareness. You can find a Feldenkrais practitioner by calling the Feldenkrais Guild of North America at (800) 775-2118 or by visiting their website at www.feldenkraisguild.com. There isn't any national organization you can contact to find an Alexander teacher, you may need to check your phone book or ask around.

Therapeutic Massage

The manipulation of soft tissues by a trained massage therapist has many benefits, including the improvement of circulation and release of knotted muscles. A skilled practitioner can focus on painful areas, encouraging the body to heal those places. Massage's pain-relieving effects are probably largely due to how relaxing it is (if it isn't, you're seeing the wrong massage therapist). It increases levels of *serotonin,* a "feel-good" neuro-transmitter, and decreases levels of stress hormones.

There are many different kinds of massage. The best types for rheumatoid arthritis patients are very gentle. Don't let a massage therapist deeply massage or otherwise manipulate inflamed joints. The best way to work on those areas is by doing your range of motion exercises.

Those with osteoarthritis can try more vigorous forms of massage, including deep tissue work, acupressure (where the therapist applies pressure to specific points), shiatsu (a Japanese form of massage that incorporates acupressure and manipulation of the joints to open up energy channels), and sports massage. Communicate closely with your massage therapist. Tell him/her about your arthritis symptoms in detail and don't be afraid to ask him/her to back off if you are in a lot of discomfort.

More and more insurers are covering massage therapy when it's warranted for pain. Physical therapists sometimes do massage as part of the treatments they deliver. Check with your insurance company to see whether it's covered on your plan.

To find a licensed massage therapist in your area, call the American Massage Therapy Association at (847) 864-0123, visit their website at www.amtamassage.org, or check your yellow pages for licensed massage therapists (LMTs). Ask family or friends whether they can recommend anyone to you.

Emotional Work and Counseling

Emotions have a lot to do with our experience of pain. (See "What Happens When You Hurt" on page 106.) This helps to explain why two people's arthritic joints, which look the same on an x-ray, may cause little or no pain in one person and debilitating pain in the other. If you are constantly wound up, stressed, and unhappy, your body's natural "feel-good" chemicals, the endorphins, are suppressed, and you feel pain more acutely.

Work with some type of counselor—whether it's a psychologist, clinical social worker, or a spiritual counselor such as a minister or rabbi—to examine any emotional, spiritual, or interpersonal issues that are causing you stress. Qualified counselors help you to keep things in perspective and give you valuable tools for coping with adversity. Once you start doing this kind of work with a counselor, you'll become more relaxed.

If all else fails, go out and rent your favorite funny movie and laugh. Laughter is an excellent stimulator of endorphin release.

Hypnosis

In a session of hypnosis, the hypnotist helps the patient reach a state of deep relaxation. While the patient is "under," the hypnotist gives verbal suggestions for changing perceptions and experiences of pain. There is plentiful clinical evidence of its effectiveness. Hypnotherapy for pain actually changes levels of biochemicals in the body that cause or intensify painful sensations.

To find a hypnotherapist, call the American Institute of Hypnotherapy at (800) 634–9766, or check your yellow pages for licensed clinical hypnotherapists.

Yoga Therapy

Yoga therapists are specially trained to teach yoga as a healing art. They learn what poses are beneficial in various conditions and teach their clients how to gain those benefits. Yoga therapy lengthens and relaxes the muscles, works the joints through their full ranges of motion, and improves circulation. The yoga therapist may also teach breathing exercises to help you control "fight-or-flight" responses to pain. Contact your local yoga studios to find out whether they have any yoga therapists on staff.

Guided Imagery

In a session of guided imagery, a specially trained therapist will talk you through some imaginary scenarios designed to help ease pain or relieve stress. If you have pain in your knee, for example, the therapist might help you imagine a gentle, healing hand massaging the joint. Once you've done the exercises with a therapist, you should be able to do them on your own at home.

If you would like to try guided imagery on your own at home, you can purchase relaxation tapes to listen to, or imagine yourself in your absolutely favorite place. For example, you could picture a tropical beach, adding all the details: warm breeze, warm sand, the sound of the waves and wafting palm hoods, the blue of the ocean, the calls of the birds, and the smell of the flowers.

HELPING YOURSELF THROUGH PAIN

Moist Heat

A long, tepid shower or bath can do wonders for relieving pain. In the shower, aim the showerhead at the places that hurt. If you have access to a Jacuzzi, relax in the tub and point the jets toward sore areas. Aromatic oils in the water can help you relax tight muscles; try myrrh oil (which is a natural pain reliever) or lavender oil.

Relaxation Techniques

When in pain, people tend to tense their muscles around the painful area. For example, if you have arthritis in your right shoulder, the muscles all around your shoulder joint, upper neck, and back will tense up. This is an unconscious way of "guarding" that area, to try to lessen the discomfort and prevent further injury. As a result of all this excess tension, other parts of the body fall out of balance and more tensions and tightness result. In the end, it can throw an already out-of-balance body even further out of whack, amplifying feelings of pain.

Relaxation techniques loosen muscles and joints. Here's a handy method for getting to a state of deep relaxation:

1. Lie on your back in a comfortable position, eyes closed. You may want to turn on some soft, meditative music.

2. Send your attention all the way down to your toes. Tense the muscles in your toes for two to four deep breaths, and then relax them. Then, send your attention to the soles of your feet, and tense and release them. Do the same with your ankles, calves, the front of your shins, knees, thighs, buttocks, belly, fingers, arms, chest, shoulders, neck, face, and scalp.

3. Lie still for a few minutes, enjoying your feeling of total relaxation.

Meditation

Meditation is in excellent way to bring yourself "into the present" and into whatever sensations are going on in your body. We spend so much energy thinking about what has already happened or what will happen, that we rarely make time to simply relax and be in this very moment.

This is especially true of people who are often in pain. The natural instinct in the face of pain is to try to escape it, to tune out and preoccupy ourselves. Much of the discomfort people in pain end up experiencing springs from their desperation to escape it. When we learn to meditate, we learn to look directly at what we are experiencing and in most cases, it isn't really as bad as we thought. A study by John Kabat-Zinn, Ph.D., included fifty-one chronic pain patients who hadn't responded to medical treatment. After a ten-week stress reduction and relaxation program, which included a meditation practice called "mindfulness meditation," 65 percent of the patients showed significant improvement. In another study, people who regularly practiced Transcendental Meditation (TM) had much milder stress responses to pain than those without meditation training.

There are many excellent teachers of meditation all over the world, so do find one that suits you and works well for you.

Magnet Therapy

This entails the use of specially designed magnets for the reduction of pain. Available in many shapes and sizes, these magnets are applied in a specific pattern around painful areas. No one is sure exactly how magnet therapy works, but it appears to offer some relief to many who use them. In some, magnets increase pain sensations at first but eventually offer total relief. Many people who use them swear by them. They can be worn for several hours at a time, but must be removed for a while each day.

Some say that magnets work by improving circulation in painful areas, flushing inflammatory and pain-stimulating biochemicals out and bringing fresh blood and nutrients in. Others guess that the magnets alter the contraction of muscle cells, or may block the passage of pain messages to the brain.

CHAPTER 9

Exercise for
Pain-Free Joints

egular exercise is one of the most important steps you can take to slow the progression of arthritis. You may not be able to run marathons, climb mountains, or swim the English Channel, but you can do a lot to keep your joints from losing their range of motion. When joints hurt, the instinctive response is to try to avoid moving them. Unless they're severely inflamed (hot, red, and swollen), you should try to move them to whatever extent you can tolerate.

For some of you, exercise is a four-letter word. When you think of exercise, you might think of donning tight-fitting workout gear to slog away on a treadmill, or some other activity involving a great deal of sweat and strain. The latest research indicates, however, that mild to moderate exercise is every bit as good for your health as intense exercise. It's actually better for you to take a pleasant walk than it is to suffer through an exercise session that you hate. The most important thing is that it's something you enjoy and that you will do consistently for the rest of your life. Whether that's walking, running, swimming, dancing, bicycling, martial arts, rock climbing, or any other mode of activity is up to you.

Maintenance of muscle strength and cardiovascular fitness, relief of pain and stiffness, and better sleep quality are some other good reasons to establish an exercise routine. Whether your arthritis is severe or mild, there is always something you can do to keep moving. By the time you finish this chapter, you'll have all the information you need to design a safe, effective exercise program for yourself.

USE IT . . . DON'T LOSE IT!

Your body is exquisitely engineered to move. When we sit for years on end at desks, in cars, or in easy chairs, the body begins to protest. If we don't take advantage of the many ways in which we can bend, squat, stretch, lift, and twist, we eventually discover that we can no longer do these things the way we used to.

The perils of a sedentary lifestyle are well known. If you don't get any exercise, your risk of having a heart attack, stroke, and cancer go up, and your chances of being overweight are much greater. Whether you're in your twenties or your eighties, it isn't too late to start exercising now. Even people in their nineties make remarkable gains in strength, flexibility, and overall health once they start an exercise program.

Moderate exercise is especially important if you want to avoid or slow the progression of osteoarthritis. Remember: Cartilage doesn't have its own blood flow and is nourished by the fluid that is pumped through it when a joint moves. Without this pumping of joint fluids, cartilage doesn't get the nutrients it needs and can't get rid of wastes and toxins. But, excessive exercise that causes repeated strain in the ankles, knees, and hips can cause osteoarthritis, so it's important to take a moderate approach. For those with rheumatoid arthritis, regular exercise is essential for maintaining joint mobility and strength, but care must be taken to avoid overdoing it or injuring weakened or inflamed joints. "Use it or lose it" is appropriate for an arthritis exercise program; "no pain, no gain" is not.

An exercise program for arthritis should include three elements: flexibility, strength, and cardiovascular fitness. First, let's talk about another element that links all three of the others: breathing.

REMEMBER TO BREATHE

I know this sounds a little bit ridiculous. How could a person forget to breathe, especially when they are exercising and need more air? Check in with your own breathing for a moment. Don't change anything, just watch. When you inhale and exhale, can you see your chest rising and falling? How about your abdomen? Place your hands on your rib cage. How much does it expand and contract with your breath?

Now, try taking a couple of deep breaths. Do your shoulders automatically hike up to your ears? Does it feel relaxing, or does it make you feel tense and light-headed to breathe deeply? Try one more thing. Go to a wall and push against it with both hands. Did you hold your breath while you were pushing?

By now, you probably have a better understanding of what it means to remember to breathe. When we don't pay attention to our breathing, it gets shallow, and the depth of our inhalations and the force of our exhalations become less. The muscles we use for breathing—the diaphragm, a large muscle below the lungs that causes them to expand, pulling air in; the intercostal and the oblique muscles, which expand the ribs wide; and even the muscles across the chest and upper back—become tense and lose their suppleness when we don't practice breathing deeply.

Being aware of the breath and learning to control it is powerfully health-promoting. When we can consciously breathe more deeply and slowly, we can relax the body through pain and stress. Holding the breath or breathing shallowly sends an alarm response through the body, causing it to make biochemicals that create tension. Taking deep, relaxed breaths soothes those responses. Deep breathing is an essential element of ancient forms of exercise such as yoga, Qigong, and Tai Chi (discussed on page 129). Meditation, the process of quieting the mind and body by focusing on the breath, can unleash the body's healing powers in ways that are just beginning to be recognized by conventional medicine. (See "A Meditation Breathing Exercise" on page 116.)

It's especially important to focus on the breath during exercise. When you strain through an exercise that hurts or is difficult, it's natural to want to hold your breath. This can cause a temporary but marked rise in blood pressure, which can be dangerous for those who have hypertension. Concentrating on breathing slowly and steadily through strength and flexibility exercises will help to make it a pleasure rather than an unpleasant chore.

CARDIOVASCULAR FITNESS

Cardiovascular exercise keeps your heart, lungs, and blood vessels strong. Attitudes about the best type of cardiovascular exercises are changing—

A Meditation Breathing Exercise

Here is a meditation exercise that will help you to focus on your breathing. Sit comfortably, with your back straight. If it's hard for you to sit straight, sit on the floor on a cushion and lean against the wall or sit in a straight-backed chair. Imagine that each of the vertebrae in your spine is stacked right on top of the one below it, and that your shoulders and arms are hanging limply from your spine. Don't slouch the shoulders forward or pinch them back. Place your hands palms up on your thighs. Tuck your chin slightly down toward your collarbone, lengthening the back of your neck. Let your sternum (the bony center of your chest) rise slightly toward your chin. Allow the space between your shoulder blades to widen. Sit quietly for a minute or two.

Now, start to focus on your inhalations and exhalations. If your nasal passages are clear, you should do both through the nose. The inhalation should start at the very base of your abdomen, causing it to expand. It then moves up to expand the lower back, the rib cage, and the sternum and upper back. Visualize it as a warm blanket of sunlight climbing up your body and draping over your shoulders. Don't let your shoulders hike up, and don't force your breath deeper than it wants to go. When you have inhaled completely, hold the breath in for two seconds.

Exhale slowly by relaxing all the muscles you used to bring the breath in. Don't force here, either; the exhale should take the same amount of time as the inhale. Exhale as much air as you can and hold the breath

we now know that it isn't necessary to sweat buckets on the treadmill or jump around in an aerobics class to keep your heart and lungs healthy. It may be as simple as walking for half an hour a day, taking a water exercise class, or doing household chores. Anything that gets you moving counts toward your daily exercise.

Arthritis patients should do some kind of cardiovascular exercise at least four days a week. One day of the week, that might mean doing household chores and walking for ten minutes to pick up something at the store. Other days, it might mean taking a half-hour walk or bicycle ride, swimming, or attending an exercise class. Mix and match activities you enjoy. Remember that the longer you go without movement, the harder it will be to get going when you finally get around to it.

there for two seconds before inhaling again. If the holding feels too uncomfortable, you can just take continuous inhalations and exhalations. If you have asthma or emphysema—diseases that can make it difficult to exhale all the air in the lungs—purse your lips through the exhalation and blow the breath out through the mouth, as though you're trying to put out a candle.

Once you get the hang of this, try doing it with your eyes closed, counting your breaths backward. On the first inhale, count fifty; on the first exhale, count forty-nine; on the next inhale, count forty-eight and so on. When you reach twenty, start only counting the inhalations. By the time you get to zero you'll feel wonderfully relaxed, alert, and invigorated.

While focusing on your breathing, allow your mind to be empty. Whenever internal chatter starts going on in your head, let it happen, but always return your attention to your breath. Don't let that internal chatter distract or frustrate you—simply let it go. If you are experiencing pain during this meditative exercise, rather than dodging away from the sensations or tensing up, fully acknowledge the places that are painful. Send your own version of healing energy into them: perhaps a caressing, massaging hand, warm rays of light, or warm water.

Try to do this meditation once each day, at whatever time you need most to relax. Some like to meditate right after rising in the morning, while others use it as a midday break. Still others meditate in the evening to unwind from the day.

If you have significant pain and stiffness in your joints, you may find that adding extra activity into your day wherever you can is the most comfortable approach. This may simply mean parking at the far end of the lot and walking, or walking on an errand rather than driving. While it's important to get your heart pumping, it's also important to listen to the messages your body is sending you. If the pain is severe, back off and rest. There's always tomorrow.

If you have arthritis in your hips, knees, or ankles, you may not be able to do weight-bearing exercise such as walking or aerobics. Your safest options under those circumstances are bicycling, swimming, or water aerobics. Stationary bicycling is a good alternative because the level of resistance can be changed to match your tolerance from day to day.

Because it alleviates some of the stress of gravity on the joints, water exercise is ideal for those who have severe arthritis in weight-bearing joints (hips, knees, ankles, and feet). Lap swimming, water jogging, and treading water are all excellent cardiovascular exercises. Accessories for water exercise are easy to find in most sporting goods stores—for example, a foam flotation belt can be worn for water jogging, and foam "weights" can be used for resistance training in the water. Plastic hand paddles and swim fins can be helpful for those with arthritic feet and hands.

Any of the range of motion, flexibility, and strengthening exercises described in this chapter can be done in the water. Many gyms, hospitals, and community pools offer water aerobics classes, where an instructor leads participants through cardiovascular and strengthening exercises in warm, shallow water, often to music. You can find water exercise classes for arthritis patients in your area by contacting your local branch of the Arthritis Foundation.

Don't worry about measuring your heart rate. Focus instead on how you are feeling. If you are breathing deeply and quickly and breaking a sweat, you're working hard enough. Try having a conversation with someone while you're exercising; if you can't speak a sentence a few words long without taking a breath, back off a little. If your joint pain is restricting you from working this hard, don't worry about it—just keep moving. Even if all you can do is work joints through their ranges of motion (see the next section for more on this), it's better than doing nothing.

It is important that you warm up before a cardiovascular workout. And after you finish, be sure to do some stretching. The range of motion and flexibility exercises described in this chapter will stretch your joints without stressing them.

Warm Up First

It's important to warm up your joints before engaging in cardiovascular exercise. Doing your range-of-motion exercises first (see pages 120–125) is a good way to accomplish this end. If you'd like to do something quicker, try the full-body warm-up routine below. Spending about five minutes on these exercises before doing your cardiovascular workout will help your joints become loose, warm, and more stable. Gently massaging joints that are especially stiff can help prepare you for exercise. Don't massage a joint that is hot and red.

You can also relieve stiffness with a warm shower or bath, or by applying a heating pad or hot water bottle. The application of heat increases blood flow and soothes away pain. If you tend to have significant pain during or after exercise, you may want to take your pain-relieving supplements before you start (see Chapter 5). If your joints are inflamed you're better off applying cold before exercise. Heat can make inflammation worse, while cold helps reduce swelling and pain. Apply an ice pack, an ice cube, or a bag of frozen peas to any inflamed joints. Remove the cold as soon as the area becomes numb; don't leave it on for more than twenty minutes. Wrapping the cold pack in a moist towel will help ease the chill. If you have any type of disorder that makes you sensitive to cold, such as vasculitis or Raynaud's phenomenon, don't apply ice. Check with your doctor or physical therapist for other options.

Full-Body Warm-up Routine

This routine is great for preparing you to do your cardiovascular exercise, and also for getting you out of bed in the morning, when stiffness can be the worst.

1. Lie on your back on your bed or on the floor. Hug one knee into your chest at a time for thirty seconds, then do some pedaling motions with your feet in the air. Perform this exercise 4–6 times.

2. Push your arms up toward the ceiling, fingers wide, and circle your wrists around several times.

3. Hug both knees into your chest, then drop them to the right for a few breaths and to the left for a few more breaths. Perform this exercise 4–6 times.

4. Roll onto your belly and come up on all fours. Round your back up toward the ceiling like a cat, then arch it so that your belly drops toward the floor. (If this hurts your wrists and hands, bend your elbows so that you're resting on your forearms. Place some folded blankets or pillows beneath your forearms to bring your back flat.) Perform this exercise 4–6 times.

Come to a seated position by dropping your hips to one side, or if you're on your bed scoot to the edge. If you're sitting on the floor, you may want to sit on a pillow or chair for exercises five through eight.

5. Tilt your head from side to side, drop your chin to your chest for a few breaths, then look back over each shoulder a few times. Perform this exercise 4–6 times.

6. Shrug your shoulders up and let them drop, then circle your shoulders back and forward a few times each. Perform this exercise 4–6 times.

7. Circle your arms as though you were swimming the crawl stroke, then circle them back as though you were doing the backstroke. Perform this exercise 4–6 times.

8. Bend and straighten your elbows. Perform this exercise 4–6 times.

9. Straighten your legs one at a time, circling your foot as you hold the leg straight. (If you are sitting on the floor, do this one lying on your back.) Perform this exercise 4–6 times.

FLEXIBILITY AND RANGE OF MOTION EXERCISE

This type of exercise is extremely important for people with arthritis. Even when you can't do any other exercise, do your best to keep up with these flexibility and range of motion movements. Range of motion exercises are designed simply to move joints in the ways they are designed to move. Flexibility exercises are designed to increase the flexibility of the tendons, ligaments, and muscles around a joint. The exercises below are a combination of both. Moving your joints—whether you do so in daily activities, or by doing flexibility and range of motion exercise—is the only way to preserve their function.

Try to push the movement of the joint as far as it will go without severe pain. Go a tiny bit beyond your comfort zone. Use your breath to help you stretch, by relaxing further into each stretch as you exhale. When you hit a place in an exercise that hurts or is extremely stiff, pause there for a full breath, allowing the exhalation to relax your joint through the sticky part. Resist the urge to tighten up.

Below are some range of motion and flexibility exercises for you to try. Focus on the ones for the joints that give you the most difficulty. Repeat each exercise three to eight times (unless otherwise indicated), moving slowly and steadily, breathing deeply, and resting between repetitions if necessary. Do the whole series twice each day. You might try doing them right after breakfast and right after dinner. If you're strapped for time, focus on the exercises for joints you have particular trouble with.

Once you learn them, you can do them anytime: waiting in line at the bank, sitting at a traffic light, or while watching TV or talking on the phone. The more often you do them, the easier they will get.

For Your Fingers

Finger Extender: Place one palm on a table and press the hand flat with the other hand.

Finger-to-Palm Stretch: Curl each finger toward your palm, one at a time, trying to touch the fingertips to the palm. Use your other hand to increase the distance each finger will stretch.

Thumb Touches: Touch each fingertip in succession to the tip of the thumb, stretching your fingers and thumb straight in between.

For Your Wrists

Inner-Wrist Stretch: Press your palms together, slightly intertwining your fingertips. Use one hand at a time to press the other hand back, stretching the inner wrist.

Back-of-Wrist Stretch: Hang one hand over the edge of a table, palm down, and use the other hand to press the fingers toward the floor, stretching the back side of the wrist.

Wrist Twists: Place both forearms on a table, palms down. Without lifting the elbows, turn the palms up, then turn them back down.

For Your Elbows

Across-the-Body Chop: Press palms together and touch them to your right shoulder. Extend the arms straight across your body, touching the hands to the outside of the left knee (if seated) or the outside of the left hip (if standing). Work to get the elbows as straight as possible. After 3–8 repetitions, reverse it.

For Your Shoulders and Chest

Shoulder Circles: Roll the shoulders forward, up, back, and down. Make the circles large and slow.

Shoulder Pivot: Hold your upper arm against your side, elbow at a right angle, forearm pointing forward, and palm facing inward. Move your hands away from each other and out to your sides, until your palms are facing front and your forearms are extending straight out from your sides. Keep your upper arms against your sides throughout.

Shoulder Opener: Clasp your hands at the base of your skull behind your neck, press your elbows back, and then bring the elbows toward one another in front of your face.

Elbow Clasp: Reach both hands behind you and grasp each wrist in the other hand. Keep your shoulders down and your chest broad. If this is comfortable, begin to walk your hands up your forearms, aiming to clasp your elbows.

Over-the-Head: Hold a light stick (or a scarf or rope drawn taut) at either end, at about chest level. There should be a distance of two to three feet between your hands. Raise the stick or scarf overhead, then return to chest level. If you can put it completely over your head and down your back, go ahead and do so.

Shoulder Pulley: Toss a rope over the top of an open door, then stand with your back to the edge of the door. Face the narrow end of the door and grab an end of the rope in each hand on either side of the door. Pull down one end at a time so that the other hand gets pulled overhead.

For Your Hips

Lying Twist: Lying on your back with knees bent, cross your right knee over the top of your left. Allow both legs to drop to the right, trying to ease them to the floor. Hold the stretch for up to one minute, then do the other side, crossing the left knee over the right and letting the legs fall to the left.

Knee Hug: Lying on your back, hug one knee at a time into the chest. You can keep the other leg bent with the foot on the floor, or extend it straight. Hold the stretch for up to a minute before switching sides.

Hip Opener: Start this one lying on your back with both knees bent, feet on the floor. Cross the right ankle just above the left knee, trying to point the right knee out to the side. Your right leg should form a triangle with your left thigh. If this feels easy, you can reach for your legs and bring them toward your chest. Hold for up to a minute. (Don't do this one if you have had a hip replacement.)

Side-Leg Scissor: Lie on your back with your legs together and knees straight. Open your legs as wide as possible, then bring them back together.

Back-Leg Extension: Stand facing a wall or chair, holding on for balance. Extend one leg straight back, keeping both legs straight and your hips square. (Imagine your hipbones have headlights in them, and you want to shine them straight ahead.) You can also do this one lying on your belly.

Boat Scoot: Sit in a straight-backed chair, with your hips all the way back in the seat. Scoot forward on the bones in your buttocks, moving one hip forward at a time, until you reach the front edge of the chair, and then scoot back.

For Your Knees

Knee Bending: Sit on the edge of a straight-backed chair and walk one foot as far beneath the chair as it will go, trying to bend the knee as much as possible. Hold for up to one minute.

Knee Straightening: Sit on a chair and place one leg on a footstool. Use the muscles in the front of the thigh to try to straighten the knee completely. If this feels easy, try leaning over the extended leg, keeping your back flat. You'll feel a powerful stretch in the back of the thigh. Hold for up to one minute.

For Your Ankles

Stair Stretch: Stand on a stair where a wall or railing is within easy reach. Turn so that your heels are at the edge of the stair, toes pointing away from the edge. Scoot the right heel back behind the left so that it hangs off the edge of the step, the ball of the foot still firmly planted. Bend the left knee, keeping the right knee straight. The right heel will press down below the level of the step, stretching the right calf muscle and ankle. Hold for up to one minute, then switch sides.

Happy Feet: Sit in a straight-backed chair, feet firmly on the floor. Lift your toes toward your nose, then place them back on the floor. Lift your heels so that the balls of your feet and your toes are pressing into the floor and return the heels to the floor. Try walking the feet to the right using this motion, then back to the left.

Ankle Circles: Sit in a chair and extend both legs forward slightly, so that the feet are off the floor. Draw big circles with your toes, both clockwise and counterclockwise.

Rolling Feet: Place a rolled up towel on the floor in front of your chair (a broom handle or rolling pin should work fine, too), so that you can place the arches of your feet on it. Roll the feet front and back to stretch and massage your arches.

For Your Neck

Half-Head Rolls: Drop your right ear toward your right shoulder, without lifting the shoulder toward the ear. Then, drop your chin down toward your chest and roll your head to the left side, dropping the ear toward the shoulder. Repeat, rolling the head back to the right, 4–8 times.

Head Turning: Turn your head to look over each of your shoulders. Inhale first, then turn the head slowly through the exhale. Inhale as you return your head to the center. Repeat 2–4 times per side.

For Your Back

Stomach Crunches: Lie on your back, knees bent, feet elevated on the seat of a chair. Use your abdominal muscles to rotate your hips slightly forward and press your lower back into the floor. This is a very small movement and can be hard to master. You can try having a friend put his or her hand beneath the small of your back, so that you can feel as though you are pressing on something.

Knee Hug: Hug one knee at a time to the chest, or hug both knees at once.

The Cobra: Lie on your belly and place your palms flat on the ground beside your shoulders. Keeping your elbows on the floor, press your head and chest up, gently arching your back. Drop your shoulders away from your ears and don't clench your buttocks. Look straight ahead.

Elbow Touch: Sit or stand and try to touch your elbows together behind you.

Cat Stretch: On all fours, arch your back toward the ceiling, then stretch the opposite way, so that your belly drops toward the ground.

STRENGTHENING EXERCISE

Strength training, also known as *resistance training,* involves pitting a muscle against some type of resistance. Going to the gym and pumping iron is resistance training. So is holding on to the back of a chair and exercising the leg muscles by squatting partway down and rising. Pushing and pulling a vacuum cleaner also qualifies. At the gym, the weights provide resistance; in the case of the squats, the weight of the body provides resistance; with the vacuuming, of course, it's the vacuum.

It's important to do some kind of resistance training. Muscle and tendon strength quickly disappear if they aren't challenged regularly. Resistance training also stimulates the bones to build themselves up. Weight-bearing exercise (walking or jogging) is universally recommended because of its bone-building effects, and it's especially important for those who can't do weight-bearing exercise to stick to a thorough strengthening program.

Don't think that being unable to hold on to weights or tubing because of arthritis makes you unable to do resistance training. There are plenty of options for you that use only your own body, the wall, or the floor as resistance. For some of the exercises described here, you can increase their intensity by using a belt, rope, inner tube, or surgical tubing. (Whatever you use should be about three feet long when laid out flat, so that it's about a foot and a half long doubled over.)

Many of the exercises recommended for strengthening fragile joints are *isometric exercises.* This means the joint is held in the same position as the muscle is tensed and released. If you were to press your palms together to work your arm muscles, you would be doing an isometric exercise. Others move the joint through its range of motion with gentle resistance.

These exercises are simple and easy to do at home without any expensive equipment. As you pull or push into the resistance, exhale smoothly. Each repetition should take you about three seconds. After a count of three, relax the muscles long enough to take a deep inhalation, then repeat. Perform eight to fifteen repetitions of each exercise, moving slowly and steadily. Do the sequence on three or four nonconsecutive days of the week. If you don't have time to do the whole series, focus on the ones for the joints that give you the most trouble.

Don't do any strengthening exercises involving any joints that are red, hot, and swollen. Only perform the range of motion and flexibility exercises for those joints until the inflammation goes down.

For Your Fingers, Hands, and Wrists

Ball Squeeze: Squeeze and release a rubber ball.

Finger-to-Thumb Press: Press the tip of each finger successively against the tip of the thumb.

Finger Lift: Put the right hand palm down on a table and place the left hand over the fingers. Lift and lower the fingers of the right hand, resisting their movement with the left. Reverse.

Finger Scoot: This exercise is especially good for those with rheumatoid arthritis, which often leads to a drifting of the fingers toward the pinky-side of the hand. Lay one hand flat on a table, fingers together and thumb spread wide. Move each finger, one at a time, toward the thumb. Use your other hand to help if needed.

Wrist lift: Place your right hand palm down on a table and place your left palm on top of it. Try to lift the right hand up from the wrist, providing resistance with the left, strengthening the top of the right wrist. Repeat with your other hand. Then, do the same exercise, but with the palm of the working hand facing up, to work the muscles on the inside of the wrist.

For Your Shoulders, Chest, and Elbows

Doorjamb Push: Stand in a doorway with the backs of your wrists against the doorjamb. Inhale, then press out steadily as you exhale for three counts. Inhale as you relax your arms.

Doorjamb Push, Part Two: Now, stand behind the doorway and reach both arms forward at shoulder level, palms facing each other. Press the arms away from one another, into the doorjamb.

Tug-of-War: Place your exercise belt around your wrists. With the upper arms against your sides and forearms pointing front, press one wrist down toward the door and the other up toward the ceiling. Hold for a count of three, exhaling, and inhale as you release.

Tug-of-War, Part Two: Try the same exercise with the arms extended straight in front of you. You'll feel this one more in the shoulders.

Bow and Arrow: Hold your exercise belt as though you were holding a bow and arrow. Pull the hands in opposite directions, exhaling as you pull and inhaling as you release. Repeat to the other side.

Prayer Press: Put your palms together in front of your chest as though you were praying. Inhale, then press the palms together steadily as you exhale.

For Your Hips and Buttocks

Squeeze and Release: Sitting in a chair with your feet on the floor, squeeze your knees together, then open them slightly. If you have a soft exercise ball for hand exercises, you can squeeze it between your knees.

Side-Leg Press: Sit in a chair with your exercise belt around both legs, just below the knees. Tie it so that it's taut when the knees are six to eight inches apart. Inhale, then press your knees away from each other through the exhale.

For Your Knees and Ankles

Leg Straightener: Sit in a chair and extend one leg straight in front of you at a time, holding for a count of three before slowly releasing it down.

Leg Bending: Stand and hold on to something for balance, feet about four inches apart. Bend one knee, bringing the heel toward the buttock, trying to keep the thighs together. Actively tuck your hips under as you do this, to avoid straining your back.

Ankle-and-Foot Strengthener: Stand with your feet four to six inches apart. Hold on to a chair or the wall if needed. Rise slowly onto your tip-toes and lower down just as slowly.

For Your Neck

Head Lift: Lie on your back with your head on a pillow. Lift your head up, bringing your chin toward your chest.

Head Press: Press the back of your head into the pillow.

For Your Stomach and Back

Stomach Crunches: See page 124.

Back Press: Sit on the floor and lean your back against a wall. Press your back into the wall for counts of three.

Bow Pose: Lie on your belly on a soft surface, with your forehead on the floor, arms by your sides, and legs straight. Inhale, and as you exhale gently raise your head, shoulders, and legs off the ground. Look toward the floor to avoid straining your neck. (Don't do this exercise if you are having lower back pain.)

TRAINING YOUR BALANCE MUSCLES

It's common for people to have trouble keeping their balance as they age. Falls that barely scratch a young person can seriously harm an older person, whose reflexes are slow to kick in. Doing balance exercises is an important part of preventing falls and preserving your sense of safety in your day-to-day activities. In fact, it isn't getting older that makes us lose our ability to balance as much as it is the lack of physical activity that usually goes along with aging. The Asian disciplines of Tai Chi, Qigong, and yoga are an excellent way to preserve balance, and classes are readily available in most urban and suburban areas. You'll find out more about them in the next section.

Some of the exercises already described are excellent for balance training. Here are a few others to add to your routine:

Walk the Line: Walk heel-to-toe along a straight line on the ground. A crack along the pavement will do, or any other straight line you can find to follow. If your balance is very poor, don't try to go heel-to-toe right away; just try to walk the line until that becomes comfortable.

One-Footed Balance: Stand near a chair or wall that you can grab if you lose your balance. Raise one foot just off the ground and balance on the other foot. If you can't do this without hanging on, try using your hand lightly to hold on, without leaning your weight onto it.

OTHER KINDS OF EXERCISE FOR ARTHRITIS

Traditional exercise forms such as yoga, Tai Chi, and Qigong are wonderful for the joints. They all share common characteristics: each promotes strength, balance, and coordination and all incorporate the use of the breath. These disciplines are often called "enlightened exercise."

Yoga originated in India, and has been practiced in many different forms for thousands of years. It combines attention to proper alignment with deep stretches and scantling poses to strengthen the large muscle groups of the lower body. Poses are usually held for several breaths. If you have arthritis, take a gentle class where you will receive plenty of attention from the instructor. There are alternate poses that can be substituted for those that hurt arthritic joints, so don't hesitate to ask the instructor for alternatives during class. Yoga classes often include meditation and end with a period of total relaxation.

Tai Chi is an Oriental martial art form. Its slow, dancelike movements are based on patterns in nature. There are actually many different kinds of Tai Chi, some of which are more challenging than others. Look for a class geared toward older people if you have arthritis. The exercises are performed from a standing position and involve a great deal of weight-shifting, turning, and pivoting on the feet, with expansive arm gestures.

Qigong is also an Oriental practice. More than 60 million people practice Qigong daily in China. It is not only a form of exercise, but also a form of meditation and a self-healing practice. Posture, breathing, and mental focus an all part of Qigong exercises.

If you are interested in trying any of these practices, you will need to seek out the guidance of a teacher in your area. Classes in all three of these practices are available in most areas of the country. Try to find an experienced teacher who can help you adapt exercises to your needs.

You may find that doing one of these practices gives you all the range-of-motion and flexibility exercise you need and other gifts you won't expect.

PACE

PACE (People with Arthritis Can Exercise) classes are offered by the Arthritis Foundation nationwide. They usually involve seated and standing exercises and are taught by qualified instructors. Contact the Arthritis Foundation in your area to find out where you can attend these classes. Exercise videos for home use are also available from the Arthritis Foundation. Call them at (800) 283–7800 or visit www.arthritis.com for information or to order.

There are many books that go into greater depth on the topic of exercise for arthritis. Check your local bookstore if you feel you'd like more information on the subject. If you're undergoing physical therapy or occupational therapy, your therapist should be able to recommend good titles.

Finding an Alternative Medicine Practitioner

There is a crisis of faith in Western medicine. Tens of millions of people every year spend more money on alternative health choices than on conventional medicine. Those who seek health want to prevent disease, not just suppress symptoms with drugs and surgery when it's too late to heal.

As people become better informed about how their dietary choices and the use of supplements and preventive medicine affects their overall health, they are likely to find themselves in disagreement with their physicians (and insurance carriers) about the best way to treat an illness. Conventional physicians have been taught that tests, drugs, and surgeries are the best medicine. Most have had barely rudimentary education about nutrition and are focused on diagnosing a disease and giving you a prescription drug to treat it.

Many people complain that their physicians don't treat them as equals, that they are only interested in writing a prescription and getting them out of the office to make room for the next patient. This isn't necessarily the physician's fault; he or she is under enormous financial pressures and time constraints. Managed care is reinforcing the "diagnose and medicate" mindset in the medical profession. Many insurance carriers won't cover alternative treatments, and most HMOs won't use physicians who embrace these methods for healing. Enjoying optimal health means going against the grain and perhaps paying out of pocket for alternative health services—at least until insurance carriers add these services to their plans. Some already offer coverage for nutritionally oriented, acupuncture, or chiropractic treatments, but they are few and far between.

To find a physician open to alternative health, including nutrition, in your area, try contacting one of these organizations:

The American College for Advancement in Medicine
23121 Verdugo Drive, Suite 204
Laguna Hills, CA 92653
(800) 532–3688
In California, call (949) 583–7666
www.acam.org

The American Holistic Medical Association
12101 Menaul Blvd., Suite C
Albuquerque, NM 87112
(505) 292-7788
www.holisticmedicine.org

Glossary

acetaminophen. A pain-relieving drug that works by blocking pain messages to the brain.

adrenaline. A hormone, also called *epinephrine,* that is released by the adrenal glands in response to stress, exercise, or strong emotion. Chronic high levels can cause insulin levels to rise, resulting in eicosanoid imbalance.

allopathic medicine. Conventional, drug- and surgery-based medicine; emphasis is on finding "magic bullets" to cure disease.

alternative medicine. Medical practices based on use of natural substances and non-invasive healing; approaches disease as a symptom of imbalance and seeks to correct it.

antioxidant. A naturally occurring substance produced in the body and in some plants that counteracts the harmful effects of free radicals. Examples include vitamins C and E, beta-carotene, and many constituents of ginger root.

arachidonic acid. A type of fatty acid found in meats and dairy products from which pro-inflammatory eicosanoids are made.

arthritis. Literally, inflammation of the joints; used in reference to over one hundred different diseases that strike connective tissues, causing joint pain, swelling, degeneration, and disability.

autoimmune disease. A condition in which the immune system loses its ability to distinguish between "self" and "not-self," and attacks the body's own tissues, causing inflammation and interfering with normal functioning. Examples include rheumatoid arthritis, ulcerative colitis, and lupus.

133

bioflavonoids. Plant compounds with powerful antioxidant properties.

bursae. Fluid-filled pads that provide cushioning between bones and between bones and skin.

candidiasis. Overgrowth of yeasts, or candida, which release toxins into the body and stimulate immune responses.

capillaries. Blood vessels with walls that are a single cell thick, through which nutrients pass to be carried away to wherever they are needed.

cartilage. The smooth protective tissue that cushions the ends of bones, reducing friction at the joints. Degeneration leads to osteoarthritis.

chondroblasts. Cells in cartilage that make protein and carbohydrate substances that fill in the spaces in collagen.

chondrocytes. Cartilage-making cells.

chyme. Food that has been partially digested in the stomach.

collagen. A fibrous protein that is the primary constituent of bone, cartilage, and connective tissue. It is the most abundant protein in the body.

collagenases. Enzymes that digest collagen.

complementary medicine. The best of both medical worlds; use of allopathic and alternative medical practices in concert with one another.

corticosteroids. Synthetic versions of cortisol, a natural anti-inflammatory hormone; commonly taken in pill form for rheumatoid arthritis and injected into joints for osteoarthritis.

cortisol. An anti-inflammatory hormone (also known as a "stress hormone") secreted by the adrenal glands in response to stress, hunger, and exercise. Chronic high levels can adversely affect eicosanoid balance.

COX. Cyclooxygenase; a type of enzyme that transforms arachidonic acid and gamma-linolenic acid (GLA) into pro-inflammatory eicosanoids.

COX-1. A form of COX that protects the lining of the gastrointestinal tract; blocking it with NSAID drugs often leads to ulcers.

COX-2. A specific form of COX enzyme that increases inflammation.

curcumin. A very potent antioxidant that has significant anti-inflammatory effects.

cytokines. Immune cells that stimulate the inflammatory response.

delayed food allergy. The intestinal immune system becomes sensitized to a food, causing inflammation; this leads to the formation of tiny leaks in the intestinal wall, allowing incompletely digested food particles into the circulation; the immune system responds, causing allergic reactions that may be subtle or obvious.

delta 5-desaturase. An enzyme that transforms activated fatty acids into eicosapentaenoic and arachidonic acids. Proper nutrition decreases delta-5 activity. This, in turn, helps decrease the formation of "bad" eicosanoids from omega-6 fats, improving eicosanoid balance.

delta 6-desaturase. An enzyme that transforms essential fats into activated fatty acids, GLA and DHGLA; this enzyme is suppressed by high cortisol and adrenaline levels caused by stress, which can disrupt eicosanoid balance.

dihomo-gamma-linolenic acid (DHGLA). An activated fatty acid that is created when delta 6-desaturase acts on linoleic acids from omega-6 oils.

disease-modifying antirheumatic drugs (DMARDs). Drugs used to treat advanced rheumatoid arthritis; work by suppressing the immune system.

duodenum. The first section of the small intestine that begins at the lower end of the stomach. It is about 25 centimeters long.

eicosanoids. Short-lived hormones that act on cells. They consist of three groups—prostaglandins, leukotrienes, and thromboxanes—which are effective in preventing blood clots, inflammation, and high blood pressure. They are important for gastrointestinal health and the health of the immune system.

eicosapentaenoic acid (EPA). The healthful fat that is created when delta 5- and delta 6-desaturase enzymes act on omega-3 oils. It is then transformed by cyclooxygenases and lipoxygenases to "good" prostaglandins and leukotrienes.

endorphins. Hormone-like substances that are natural painkillers and mood enhancers. They are found primarily in the brain.

endotoxins. Toxins formed within the body in the natural course of its day-to-day functions

essential fatty acids (EFAs). Fatty acids necessary for health that are obtained only through diet. Omega-3 and omega-6 are the two types.

exotoxins. Toxins such as prescription drugs, chemicals found in the environment, and artificial food additives, preservatives, which come into the body from outside.

free radicals. An atom or group of atoms with at least one unpaired electron, making it highly unstable. Free radicals join readily with other substances and can cause damage at the cellular level. They are the result of normal metabolism, as well as the result of exposure to radiation, pollutants, and the inflammatory process. They are blocked by antioxidants.

fructooligosaccharides. The preferred food of probiotic bacteria.

gamma-linolenic acid (GLA). Linolenic acids from omega-6 fats that have been acted upon by delta 6–desaturase enzyme.

gastric. Having to do with the stomach.

gingerols. The most potent constituents of ginger oleoresin.

glycosaminoglycans (GAGs). Sugar and protein molecules that link together to form proteoglycans; glucosamine sulfate is an example of a GAG.

Helicobacter pylori (H. pylori). Bacteria that grows in the mucus-secreting cells of the stomach lining. It is a common cause of gastritis, ulcer, heartburn, and chronic indigestion.

hyaluronic acid. A substance in synovial fluid; gives fluid its viscosity and shock-absorbing quality. It is destroyed by free radicals that are created during inflammation.

hydrochloric acid (HCl). The strong acid secreted by the stomach to aid in the digestion of food.

inflammation. The body's immune response to injury, or to invasion by infectious agents or toxins; characterized by heat, swelling, redness, and pain.

interleukins. Part of the immune system that helps regulate an immune response. They play a key role in regulating inflammation.

isometric exercise. Working muscles against resistance that does not move; for example, pushing against an immovable object to exercise the arm muscles.

leaky gut syndrome. A condition in which food sensitivities lead to inflammation in the small intestine, causing small holes to form. Partially digested food particles and toxins pass through these leaks and enter the bloodstream, eventually compromising the body's immune system. Leaky gut is associated with a number of autoimmune conditions such as asthma, chronic fatigue, and arthritis.

leukotriene. A type of eicosanoid that helps regulate inflammation, immunity, mucous secretion, and muscle contraction.

lipoxygenases. A group of enzymes responsible for the formation of "good" and "bad" leukotrienes.

lymphocytes. Immune cells; important in regulating the inflammatory process.

macronutrients. Carbohydrates, protein, and fats; the calorie-containing parts of the food we eat.

micronutrients. Vitamins, minerals, and other phytochemicals that have nutritional value but contain no calories.

motility. The speed at which food moves through the digestive tract.

natural killer (NK) cell. Type of immune cell that can kill certain cancer cells.

nitric oxide. A chemical made in the body that relaxes muscles in blood vessel walls, allowing them to open.

nutraceuticals. Natural therapeutic products that contain substances that exist in nature.

nightshade vegetables. A family of vegetables that includes tomatoes, potatoes, red and green peppers, eggplant, tobacco, and cayenne pepper that have been shown to exacerbate arthritis.

nonsteroidal anti-inflammatory drugs (NSAIDs). Any of a class of over-the-counter or prescription drugs that are commonly used to relieve mild to moderate pain.

noriceptors. Nerve endings that are located in the skin and throughout the internal organs, joints, and bones that sense different types or pain.

oleoresin. The sticky part of the ginger rhizome that contains most of its active ingredients.

omega-3 fats. Essential fats found in fish oils and certain vegetable oils, including canola and flaxseed. They are the raw material for "good" eicosanoids.

omega-6 fats. Essential fats found in unsaturated oils, such as black currant, borage, evening primrose, grapeseed, sesame seed, and soybean; also present in raw nuts, seeds, and legumes. They are the raw material for both "good" and "bad" eicosanoids.

orthomolecular medicine. The use of high doses of nutrients found in foods to treat illness.

osteoarthritis. The most common form of arthritis in which the cartilage that cushions joints begins to wear. It is believed to be caused primarily by wear and tear.

oxidation. A chemical reaction in which oxygen reacts with another substance, often resulting in some type of spoilage. This process causes free radicals.

pepsin. An enzyme secreted in the stomach that breaks down proteins during digestion. Most ulcer drugs decrease pepsids action, adversely affecting digestion.

peristalsis. Rhythmic muscular contractions of the gastrointestinal tract that move food along during the digestive process.

phytochemicals. Any one of a number of substances found in plants that have various health-promoting properties, including protection against certain types of cancer.

platelets. Components of blood responsible for clotting.

probiotics. "Friendly" bacteria that live in the gastrointestinal, genital, and urinary tracts; manufacture vitamins and keep "unfriendly" bacteria and yeasts from becoming overgrown. They manufacture B vitamins, aid in the digestive process, and neutralize toxins and carcinogens.

prostacyclin. A "good" prostaglandin that maintains proper blood fluidity and dilates blood vessels. Celebrex, commonly prescribed for arthritis, suppresses its formation.

prostaglandin. Type of eicosanoid that affects pain sensations, inflammation, body temperature, the constriction and expansion of blood vessels, blood clotting and the health of the stomach lining. It also plays a key role in regulating body temperature, expanding and contracting blood vessels, and maintaining proper blood fluidity and healthy stomach lining.

proteoglycans. Made of glycosaminoglycans (GAGs); weave through collagen fibers to form connective tissue.

putrefactive bacteria. "Bad" bacteria, such as *E. coli* and clostridium, that can become overgrown and toxic to the body if "good" bacterial populations decrease.

rheumatoid arthritis. An autoimmune disorder in which the immune system mistakenly attacks the body's own tissues, causing chronic inflammation, pain, and joint swelling.

rhizome. Rootlike part of a plant that is able to bud and grow if split and replanted.

serotonin. A neurotransmitter that is important for regulating a number of functions, including mood, relaxation, sleep, and concentration. Because of its interactions with platelets and substance P, it may play a role in causing migraine headaches.

specificity. Describes the ability of a drug to affect one body process without affecting any others.

substance P. A chemical produced in the body that stimulates the sensation of pain.

synergistic ingredients. Plant substances that help the active ingredients perform their functions.

thromboxane synthetase. An enzyme needed to make thromboxanes. Increased levels suppress the formation of endorphins, while decreased levels encourage it.

thromboxanes. Eicosanoids responsible for the regulation of blood clotting and pain responses.

toxin. Any substance that can do damage to living tissue; *exotoxins* come into the body from outside, while *endotoxins* are formed within the body in the natural course of its' day-to-day functions.

transit time. The amount of time necessary for the digestive process to take place, from start to finish.

tumor necrosis factor. A cancer-fighting arm of the immune system, thought to be involved in the causes of both osteoarthritis and rheumatoid arthritis.

zingibain. Protein-digesting enzyme found in ginger root.

References

Aaseth, J., Haugen, M., and Forre, O., "Rheumatoid arthritis and metal compounds–perspectives on the role of oxygen radical detoxification." *Analyst* 123(l) (January 1998): 3–6.

Adderly, B., *The Arthritis Cure Fitness Solution.* (Washington, D.C.: Regnery Publishing, 1999).

Ahmed, R. S., and Shama, S. B., "Biochemical studies on combined effects of garlic (Allium sativum Linn) and ginger (Zingiber officinale Rosc.) in albino rats." *Indian Journal of Experimental Biology* 35(8) (August 1997): 841–43.

Alaaedine, N., et al., "Inhibition of tumor necrosis factor alpha-induced prostaglandin E2 production by the anti-inflammatory cytokines interleukin-4, interleukin-10, and interleukin-13 in synovial fibroblasts: distinct targeting in the signaling pathways." *Arthritis and Rheumatism* 42(4) (April 1999): 710–18.

Alexander, J. W., "Immunonutrition: the role of omega-3 fatty acids." *Nutrition* 14(7–8) (July/August 1998): 627–33.

al-Yahya, M. A., et al., "Gastroprotective activity of ginger zingiber officinale rosc., in albino rats." *American Journal of Chinese Medicine* 17(1–2) (1989): 51–56.

Amin, A. R., and Abramson, S. B., "The role of nitric oxide in articular cartilage breakdown in osteoarthritis." *Current Opinion in Rheumatology* (10 May 1998): 263–68.

Ammon, H. P., et al., "Mechanism of anti-inflammatory actions of curcumin and boswellic acids." *Journal of Ethnopharmacology* 38(2–3) (March 1993): 113–19.

141

Arfeen, Z., et al., "A double-blind randomized controlled trial of ginger for the prevention of postoperative nausea and vomiting." *Anaesthesia and Intensive Care* 23(4) (August 1995): 449–52.

Astin, J. A., "Stress reduction through mindfulness meditation: effects on psychological symptomatology, sense of control, and spiritual experiences." *Psychotherapy and Psychosomatics* 66(2) (1997): 97–106.

Attur, M. G., et al., "Autocrine production of IL-1 B by human osteoarthritis-affected cartilage and differential regulation of endogenous nitric oxide, IL-6, prostaglandin E2 and IL-8." *Proceedings of the Association of American Physicians* 110 (January/February 1998): 1, 65–72.

Austin, S., "Double-blinded evidence supports cetyl myristoleate." *Quarterly Review of Natural Medicine* (Winter 1997): 315–16.

Austin, S., "The confusion over chondroitin." *Quarterly Review of Natural Medicine* (Summer 1997): 125–26.

Backon, J., "Ginger and carbon dioxide as thromboxane synthetase inhibitors: potential utility in treating peptic ulceration." *Gut* 28 (1987): 1323.

Backon, J., "Ginger: inhibition of thromboxane synthetase and stimulation of prostacyclin: relevance for medicine and psychiatry." *Medical Hypotheses* 20(3) (July 1986): 271–78.

Backon, J., "Mechanism of analgesic effect of clonidine in the treatment of dysmenorrhea." *Medical Hypotheses* 36(3) (November 1991): 223–24.

Bang, B., et al., "Reduced 25–hydroxyvitamin D levels in primary Sjögren's syndrome: correlations to disease manifestations." *Scandinavian Journal of Rheumatology* 28(3) (1998): 180–83.

Barclay, T. S., Tsourounis, C., and McCart, G. M., "Glucosamine." *Annals of Pharmacotherapy* 32(5) (May 1998): 574–79.

Bassleer, C., Rovati, L., and Franchimont, P., "Stimulation of proteoglycan production by glucosamine sulfate in chondrocytes isolated from human osteoarthritic articular cartilage in vitro." *Osteoarthritis and Cartilage* 6(6) (November 1998): 427–34.

Bates, C. J., "Proline and hydroxyline excretion and vitamin C status in elderly human subjects." *Clinical Science and Molecular Medicine* 52 (1977): 525–43.

Batson, G., "Alleviating arthritis pain and discomfort: how the Alexander

Technique can help." A Web page provided as a service by Alexander Technique Nebraska and the Ontario Centre for the Alexander Technique.

Belanger, A. Y., "Physiological evidence for an endogenous opiate-related pain-modulating system and its relevance to TENS: a review." *Physiotherapy Canada* 37(3) (1985): 163–68.

Belch, J. F., et al., "Effects of altering dietary essential fatty acids on requirements for nonsteroidal anti-inflammatory drugs in patients with rheumatoid arthritis: a double-blind placebo controlled study." *Annals of Rheumatic Diseases* 47 (1988): 96–104.

Bennett, W. M. "Drug-related renal dysfunction in the elderly." *Geriatric Nephrology and Urology* 9(1) (1999): 21–25.

Berman, B. M., et al., "Efficacy of traditional Chinese acupuncture in the therapy of symptomatic knee osteoarthritis: a pilot study." *Osteoarthritis and Cartilage* 3(2) (June 1995): 139–42.

Berry, E. M., and Hirsch, J., "Does dietary linolenic acid influence blood pressure?" *American Journal of Clinical Nutrition* 44 (1986): 336–40.

Bhandari, U., Sharma, N., and Zafar, R., "The protective action of ethanolic ginger (Zingiber officinale) extract in cholesterol fed rabbits." *Journal of Ethnopharmacology* 61(2) (June 1998): 167–71.

Birch, S., et al., "Acupuncture in the therapy of pain." *Journal of Alternative and Complementary Medicine* 2(1) (Spring 1996): 101–24.

Bjarnsason, I., "Forthcoming NSAIDs: are they really devoid of side effects?" *Italian Journal of Gastroenterology and Hepatology* 31 Suppl (1999): 927–36.

Bjorkman, D. J., "The effect of aspirin and nonsteroidal anti-inflammatory drugs on prostaglandins." *American Journal of Medicine* 105(b) (27 July 1998): 8S-12S.

Bland, J. H., and Cooper, S. M., "Osteoarthritis: a review of the cell biology involved and evidence for reversibility. Management rationally related to known genesis and pathophysiology." *Seminars in Arthritis and Rheumatism* 14 (1984): 106–33.

Bland, J. H., *Intestinal Toxicity and Inner Cleansing*. (New Canaan, CT: Keats Publishing, 1991).

Blond, J. P., and Lemarchel, P., "A study on the effect of alpha-linolenic acid on the desaturation of dihomogamma-linolenic acids using rat liver homogenates." *Reproductive Nutrition Development* 24 (1984): 1–10.

Bordia, A., Verma, S. K., and Srivastava, K. C., "Effect of ginger (Zingiber officinale Rosc.) and fenugreek (Trigonella foenumgraecum L.) on blood lipids, blood sugar and platelet aggregation in patients with coronary artery disease." *Prostaglandins, Leukotrienes, Essential Fatty Acids* 56(5) (May 1997): 379–84.

Borkman, M., et al., "The relationship between insulin sensitivity and the fatty acid composition of skeletal muscle phospholipids." *New England Journal of Medicine* 328 (1993): 238–44.

Bostrom, C., et al., "'Effect of static and dynamic shoulder rotator exercises in women with rheumatoid arthritis: a randomized comparison of impairment, disability, handicap, and health." *Scandinavian Journal of Rheumatology* 27(4) (1998): 281–90.

Brenner, R. R., "Nutritional and hormonal factors influencing desaturation of essential fatty acids." *Progressive Lipid Research* 20 (1982): 41–48.

Brooks, P. M., and Potter, S. R., "NSAID and arthritis–help or hindrance?" *Journal of Rheumatology* 9 (1982): 3–5.

Brown, D., Gaby, A., and Reichert, R., "Clinical applications of natural medicine: migraine." *Quarterly Review of Natural Medicine* (Summer 1997): 147–58.

Buckwalter, J. A., "Osteoarthritis and articular cartilage use, disuse, and abuse: experimental studies," *Journal Of Rheumatology* Suppl 43 (February 1995): 13–5.

Burton, T. M., and Langreth, R., "Initial sales surge for monsanto arthritis drug." *The Wall Street Journal* (27 January 1999).

Calder, P. C., "n-3 polyunsaturated fatty acids -and cytokine production in health and disease." *Annals of Nutrition and Metabolism* 41(4) (1997): 203–34.

Cao, Z. F., et al., "Scavenging effects of ginger on superoxide anion and hydroxyl radical." *Chung Kuo Chung Yoa Tsa Chih* 18(12) (December 1993): 750–51, 764.

Caughey, D. E., et al., "Perna canaliculus in the treatment of rheumatoid arthritis." *European Journal of Rheumatology and Inflammation* 6(2) (1983): 197–206.

Chou, C. T., Uksila, J., and Toivanen, P., "Enterobacterial antibodies in Chinese patients with rheumatoid arthritis and ankylosing spondylitis." *Clinical and Experimental Rheumatology* 16(2) (March/April 1998): 161–64.

Christensen, B. V., et al., "Acupuncture treatment of severe knee osteoarthrosis: a long-term study." *Acta Anaesthesiologica Scandinavia* 36(6) (August 1992): 519–25.

Cichoke, A. J., "Treating rheumatoid arthritis with enzymes. *Townsend Letter for Doctors and Patients* (January 1996): 32–34.

Cohen, A., and Goldman, J., "Bromelain therapy in rheumatoid arthritis." *Pennsylvania Medical Journal* 67 (1964): 27–30.

Cohen, D., *Arthritis: Stop Suffering, Start Moving*. (New York, NY: Walter and Company, 1995).

Comstock, G. W., et al., "Serum concentrations of alpha tocopherol, beta-carotene, and retinol preceding the diagnosis of rheumatoid arthritis and systemic lupus erythematosus." *Annals of Rheumatic Diseases* 56 (1997): 323–25.

Cooper, K. *Arthritis; Your Complete Exercise Guide*. (Champaign, IL: Cooper Clinic and Research Institute Fitness Series, Human Kinetics Publishing, 1992).

Coulston, A. M., Liu, G. C., and Reaven, G. M., "Plasma, glucose, insulin and lipid responses to high-carbohydrate, low-fat diets in normal humans." *Metabolism* 32 (1983): 52–56.

Cranton, E., and Fryer, W., *Resetting the Clock*. (New York, NY: M. Evans and Company, 1996).

Cryer, B., et al., "Cyclooxygenase-1 and cyclooxygenase-2 selectivity of widely used nonsteroidal anti-inflammatory drugs." *American Journal of Medicine* 104(5) (May 1998): 413–21.

Cunnane, S. C., et al., "Alpha-linolenic acid in humans: direct functional role or dietary precursor?" *Nutrition* 7 (1991): 437–39.

DaCamara, C. C., and Dowless, G. V., "Glucosamine sulfate for osteoarthritis." *Annals of Pharmacotherapy* 32(5) (May 1998): 580–87.

Darlington, L. G., Ramsey, N. W., and Mansfield, J. R., "Placebo-controlled, blind study of dietary manipulation in rheumatoid arthritis." *Lancet* i (1986): 236–38.

Das, U. N., "Beneficial effect of eicosapentaenoic and docosahexaenoic acids in the management of systemic lupus erythematosus and its relationship to the cytokine network." *Prostaglandins, Leukotrienes, and Essential Fatty Acids* 51(3) (September 1994): 207–13.

Deal, C. L., and Moskowitz, R. W., "Nutraceuticals as therapeutic agents in osteoarthritis. The role of glucosamine, chondroitin sulfate, and collagen hydrolysate." *Rheumatic Disease Clinics of North America* 25(2) (May 1999): 379–95.

DeKeyser, F., et al., "Bowel inflammation and the spondyloarthropathies." *Rheumatic Disease Clinics of North America* 24(4) (November 1998): ix–x, 785–813.

DeMarco, D. M., Santoli, D., and Zurier, R. B., "Effects of fatty acids on proliferation and activation of human synovial compartment lymphocytes." *Journal of Leukocyte Biology* 56(5) (November 1994): 612–15.

Diehl, W., and May, E. L., "Cetyl myristoleate isolated from Swiss albino mice: an apparent protective agent against adjuvant arthritis in rats." *Journal of Pharmaceutical Science* 83(3) (March 1994): 296–99.

Dolby, V., "Ouch! Nutritional approaches to help you say 'aaahh." *Better Nutrition* (May 1998): 18.

Domangue, B. B., et al., "Biochemical correlates of hypnoanalgesia in arthritic pain patients." *Journal of Clinical Psychiatry* 46(6) (June 1985): 235–38.

Edmonds, S.. E., et al., "Putative analgesic activity of repeated oral doses of vitamin E in the treatment of rheumatoid arthritis: results of a prospective placebo-controlled, double-blind trial." *Annals of Rheumatic Disease* 56(11) (November 1997): 649–55.

Fawzy, A. A., Vishwanath, B. S., and Franson, R. C., "Inhibition of human non-pancreatic phospholipases A2 by retinoids, and flavonoids. Mechanism of action." *Agents and Actions* 25(3–4) (December 1988): 394–400.

Feldman, M., et al., "Effects of aging and gastritis on gastric acid and pepsin secretion in humans: a prospective study." *Gastroenterology* 110(4) (April 1996): 1043–52.

Fischer, S. M., "Prostaglandins and cancer." *Frontiers in Bioscience 2*, 2 (1 October 1997): 482–500.

Flynn, D., et al., "Inhibition of human neutrophil 5–lipoxygenase activity by gingerdione, shogaol, capsaicin and related pungent compounds." *Prostaglandins, Leukotrienes, and Medicine* 24 (1986): 195–98.

Fort, J., "Celecoxib, a COX-2–specific inhibitor: the clinical data." *American Journal of Orthopedics* 28(3 Suppl) (March 1999): 8–12.

Fosslien, E., "Adverse effects of nonsteroidal anti-inflammatory drugs on the gastrointestinal system." *Annals of Clinical Laboratory Science* 28(2) (March/April 1998): 67–81.

Fretland, D. J., "Pharmacological activity of the second generation leukotriene B4 receptor antagonist, SC53228: effects on colonic inflammation and hepatic function in rodents." *Inflammation* 19(5) (October 1995): 503–15.

Fries, J. F., et al., "Toward an epidemiology of gastropathy associated with nonsteroidal and anti-inflammatory drug use." *Gastroenterology* 96 (1989): 647–55.

Frondosa, C. O., et al., "Expression of pro-inflammatory IL1 and TNF-alpha by osteoarthritic chondrocytes is altered in response to mechanical stress." Orthopaedic Research Society, 45th Annual Meeting, Anaheim, CA, February 1–4, 1999.

Fuhrman, J., *Fasting–and Eating–for Health.* (St. Martin's Griffin, New York, NY: 1998).

Fulder, S., *The Ginger Book.* (Garden City Park, NY: Avery Publishing Group, 1996).

Fung, H. B., and Kirschenbaum, H. L., "Selective cyclooxygenase-2 inhibitors for therapy of arthritis." *Clinical Therapeutics* 21(7) (July 1999): 1131–57.

G. D. Searle and Company. Press release on Celebrex. November 12, 1998.

Gabor, M., et al., "Effects of benzopyrone derivatives on simultaneously induced croton oil ear oedema and carageenan paw oedema in rats." *Acta Physiologica Hungaria* 65(2) (1985): 235–40.

Galland, L., "Nutrition and candidiasis." *Journal of Orthomolecular Psychiatry* 15 (1985): 50–60.

Garfinkel, M. S., "Yoga-based intervention for carpal tunnel syndrome: a randomized trial." *JAMA* 280(18) (11 November 1998): 1601–03.

Garfinkel, M. S., et al., "Evaluation of a yoga-based regimen for treatment of osteoarthritis of the hands." *Journal of Rheumatology* 12 (21 December 1994): 2341–43.

Geis, G. S. "Update on clinical developments with celecoxib, a new specific COX-2 inhibitor: what can we expect?" *Journal of Rheumatology* 26 Suppl 56 (April 1999): 31–36.

Geusens, P., et al., "Long term effect of omega-3 fatty acid supplementation in active rheumatoid arthritis: a 12–month, double-blind controlled study." *Arthritis and Rheumatism* 37(6) (1994): 824–29.

Glick, L., "Deglycyrrhizinated licorice in peptic ulcer." *Lancet* ii (1982): 817.

Golan, R., *Optimal Wellness*. (New York, NY: Ballantine Books, 1995).

Goodrick, C. L., et al., "Effects of intermittent feeding upon growth, activity and lifespan in rats allowed voluntary exercise." *Experimental Aging Research* 9 (1983): 1477–94.

Goso, Y., et al., "Effects of traditional herbal medicine of gastric mucin against ethanol-induced gastric injury in rats." *Comparative Biochemistry and Physiology* 11 (13C) (1996): 17–21.

Govindarajan, V. S., "Ginger chemistry, technology, and quality evaluation." *CRC Critical Reviews of Food Sciences and Nutrition* 17 (1982): 1–258.

Guan, Z., and Zhang, J., "Effects of acupuncture on immunoglobulins in patients with asthma and rheumatoid arthritis." *Journal of Traditional Chinese Medicine* 15(2) (June 1995): 102–05.

Guslandi M., and Ballarin, E., "Assessment of the 'mucus-bicarbonate' barrier in the stomach of patients with chronic gastric disorders." *Clinica Chimica Acta* 144(2–3) (29 December 1984): 133–36.

Guslandi, M., Pellegrini, A., and Sorghi, M., "Gastric mucosal defenses in the elderly." *Gerontology* 45(4) (July 1999): 206–08.

Gwen, R. N., Ellert, B. S. N., and Koehler, B., *The Arthritis Exercise Book: Gentle Joint by Joint Exercise to Keep You Flexible and Independent* (Lincolnwood, IL: NTC/Contemporary Publishers, 1990).

Haanen, H. C., et al., "Controlled trial of hypnotherapy in the treatment of refractory fibromyalgia." *Journal of Rheumatology* 18(1) (January 1991): 72–75.

Hafstrom, I., et al., "Effects of fasting on disease activity, neutrophil function, fatty acid, composition, leukotriene biosynthesis in patients with rheumatoid arthritis." *Arthritis and Rheumatism* 31 (1988): 585.

Hamilton, L. C., et al., "Synergy between cyclooxygenase-2 induction and arachidonic acid supply in vivo: consequences for nonsteroidal anti-inflammatory drug efficacy." *FASEB Journal* 13(2) (February 1999): 245–51.

Hansen, T. M., et al., "Treatment of rheumatoid arthritis, with prostaglandin El precursors cis-linoleic acid and gamma-linoleic acid." *Scandinavian Journal of Rheumatology* 12(2) (1983): 85–8.

Hasenohrl, R. U., et al., "Anxiolytic-like effect of combined extracts of Zingiber officinale and ginkgo biloba in the elevated plus-maze." *Pharmacology Biochemistry, and Behavior* 53(2) (February 1996): 271–75.

Hashim, S., et al., "Modulatory effects of essential oils from spices on the formation of DNA adduct by aflatoxin B I in vitro." *Nutrition and Cancer* 21(2) (1994): 169–75.

Heller, A., et al., "Lipid mediators in inflammatory disorders." *Drugs* 55(4) (April 1998): 487–96.

Hill, E. G., et al., "Perturbation of the metabolism of essential fatty acids by dietary partially hydrogenated vegetable oil." *Proceedings of the National Academy of Sciences* USA 79 (1982): 953–57.

Hoffer, A., "Treatment of arthritis by nicotinic acid and nicotinamide." *Canadian Medican Association Journal* 81 (1959): 235–39.

Hojgaard, L., Mertz-Nielsen, A., and Rune, S. J., "Peptic ulcer pathophysiology: acid, bicarbonate, and mucosal function." *Scandinavian Journal of Gastroenterology* Suppl 216 (1996): 10–15.

Horn, C., "13 Ways to Wipe Out Pain." *Natural Health* (January/February 1999): 129–39.

Horrobin, D. F., et al., "The regulation of prostaglandin El formation: a candidate for one of the fundamental mechanisms involved in the action of vitamin C." *Medical Hypotheses* 5(8) (1979): 849–58.

Huang, Q. R., et al., "Anti-5–hydroxytryptamine 3 effect of galanolactone, diterpenoid isolated from ginger." *Chemical Pharmacy Bulletin* 39(2) (February 1991): 397–99.

Hurley, M. V., "The role of muscle weakness in the pathogenesis of osteoarthritis." *Rheumatic Disease Clinics of North America* 25(2) (May 1999): vi, 283–98.

Jacob, S. W., Lawrence, R. M., and Zucker, M., *The Miracle of MSM: The Natural Solution for Pain.* (New York, NY: G. P. Putnam's Sons, 1999).

Jefferies, W. M., "The etiology of rheumatoid arthritis." *Medical Hypotheses* 51(2) (August 1998): 111–14.

Jefferies, W. M., *Safe Uses of Cortisol.* (Springfield, IL: Charles C. Thomas, Publisher, 1996).

Jobin, C., et al., "Curcumin blocks cytokine-mediated NF-kappa-B activation and pro-inflammatory gene expression by inhibiting inhibitory factor 1–kappa-B kinase activity." *Journal of Immunology* 163(6) (15 September 1999): 3474–483.

Johnson, M. I., Ashton, C. H., and Thompson, J. W., "The clinical use of TENS." *Journal of Orthopedic Medicine* 14(1) (1992): 3–12.

Jonas, W. B., Rapoza, C. P., and Blair, W. F., "The effect of niacinimide on osteoarthritis: a pilot study." *Inflammation Research* 45 (1996): 330–34.

Jones, G., et al., "Allelic variation in the vitamin D receptor, lifestyle factors and lumbar spinal degenerative disease." *Annals of Rheumatic Disease* 57(2) (February 1998): 94–99.

Kabat-Zinn, J., "An outpatient program in behavioral medicine for chronic pain patients based on the practice of mindfulness meditation: theoretical considerations and preliminary results." *General Hospital Psychiatry* 4(1) (April 1982): 33–47.

Kabat-Zinn, J., "The clinical use of mindfulness meditation for the self-regulation of chronic pain." *Journal of Behavioral Medicine* 8(2) (June 1985): 163–90.

Kaplan-Machlis, B., et al., "The cyclooxygenase-2 inhibitors: safety and effectiveness," *Annals of Pharmacotherapy* 33(9) (September 1999): 979–88.

Katiyar, S. K., Agarwal, R., and Mukhtar, H., "Inhibition of tumor promotion in SENCAR mouse skin by ethanol extract of Zingiber officinale rhizome." *Cancer Research* 56(5) (1 March 1996): 1023–30.

Kelley, D. S., "Alpha-linolenic acid and immune response." *Nutrition* 8 (1992): 215–17.

Kenyon, J. N., "Food sensitivity, a search for underlying causes: case study of 12 patients." *Acupuncture and Electrotherapy Research* 110 (1986): 1–13.

Keplinger, K., et al., "Uncaria tomentosa (Wild) DC–ethnomedicinal use and new pharmacological, toxicological and botanical results." *Journal of Ethnopharmacology* 64(1) (January 1999): 23–34.

Kheir-Eldin, A. A., et al., "Biochemical changes in arthritic rats under the influence of vitamin E." *Agents and Actions* 36(3–4) (July 1992): 300–05.

Kjeldsen-Kragh, J., et al., "Dietary omega-3 fatty acid supplementation and naproxen treatment in patients with rheumatoid arthritis. "*Journal of Rheumatology* 19(10) (October 1992): 15, 31–36.

Kose, K., et al., "Plasma selenium levels in rheumatoid arthritis." *Biological Trace Element Research* 53(1–3) (Summer 1996): 51–56.

Kremer, J., et al., "Effects of manipulation of dietary fatty acids on clinical manifestation of rheumatoid arthritis." *Lancet* i (1985): 184–87.

Kremer, J. M., et al., "Effects of high-dose fish oil on rheumatoid arthritis after stopping NSAIDs: clinical and immune correlates." *Arthritis and Rheumatism* 38(8) (1995): 1107–14.

Kroker, G. E., et al., "Fasting and rheumatoid arthritis: a multi-center study." *Clinical Ecology* 2(3) (1984): 137–144.

Krystal, G., et al., "Stimulation of DNA synthesis by ascorbate in cultures of articular chondrocytes." *Arthritis and Rheumatism* 25 (1982): 525–43.

Kumakura, S., Yamashita, M., and Tsurufuji, S., "Effect of bromelain on kaolin-induced inflammation in rats," *European Journal of Pharmaology* 150 (10 June 1988): 295–301.

LaCorte, R., et al., "Prophylaxis and therapy of NSAID-induced gastrointestinal disorders." *Drug Safety* 20(6) (June 1999): 527–43.

Lane, N. E., et al., "Serum vitamin D levels and incident changes of radiographic hip osteoarthritis: a longitudinal study. Study of Osteoporosis Fractures Research Group." *Arthritis and Rheumatism* 42(5) (May 1999): 854–60.

Larsson, P., et al., "A vitamin D analogue (MC 1288) has immunomodulatory properties and suppresses collagen-induced arthritis (CIA) without causing hypercalcemia." *Clinics in Experimental Immunology* 114(2) (November 1998): 277–83.

Lau, C. S., Morley, K. D., and Belch, J. J., "Effects of fish oil supplementation on nonsteroidal anti-inflammatory drug requirement in patients with mild rheumatoid arthritis—a double-blind, placebo-controlled study." *British Journal of Rheumatology* 32(11) (November 1993): 982–89.

Lee, E., and Surj, Y.J., "Induction of apoptosis in HL-60 cells by pungent vanilloids, [6]-gingerol and [6]-paradol." *Cancer Letters* 134(2) (25 December 1998): 163–68.

Leffler, C. T., et al., "Glucosamine, chondroitin, and manganese ascorbate for degenerative joint disease of the knee or low back: a randomized, double-blind, placebo-controlled pilot study." *Milano Medicine* 164(2) (February 1999): 85–91.

Lipsky, R. E., "Specific COX-2 inhibitors in arthritis, oncology, and beyond: where is the science headed?"*Journal of Rheumatology* 26 (56 Suppl) (April 1999): 25–30.

Liu, X., et al., "Effect of acupuncture and point-injection treatment on immunologic function in rheumatoid arthritis." *Journal of Traditional Chinese Medicine* 13(3) (September 1993): 174–78.

Lumb, A. B., "Effect of dried ginger on human platelet function." *Thrombosis and Haemostasis* 710 (January 1994): 110–11.

Machtey, I., and Ouaknine, L., "Tocopherol in osteoarthritis: a controlled pilot study." *Journal of the American Geriatric Society* 25(7) (1978): 328.

Madrid, A. D., and Barnes, S. H., "A hypnotic protocol for eliciting physical changes through suggestions of biochemical responses." *American Journal of Clinical Hypnotism* 34(2) (October 1991): 122–28.

Mahmud, Z., and Ali, S. M., "Role of vitamin A and E in spondylosis." *Bangladesh Medical Research Council Bulletin* 18(1) (April 1992): 47–59.

Manning, A., "Arthritis enzyme linked to diseases." *USA Today* (5 August 1998).

Mantizioris, E., et al., "Dietary substitution with alpha-linolenic acid-rich vegetable oil increases eicosapentaenoic acid concentrations in tissues." *American Journal of Clinical Nutrition* 59 (1994): 1304–09.

Marshall, K. W., "Practical implications of cyclooxygenase 2–specific inhibitors in orthopedics." *American Journal of Orthopedics* 28(3 Suppl) (March 1999): 19–21.

Mascob, N., et al., "Ethnopharmacological investigations on ginger (Zingiber officinale)." *Journal of Ethnopharmacology* 27 (1989): 129–40.

Masi, A. T., Chatterton, R. T., and Aldag, J. C., "Perturbations of hypothalamic-pituitary-gonadal axis and adrenal androgen functions in rheumatoid arthritis: an odyssey of hormonal relationships to the disease." *Annals of the New York Academy of Sciences* 876 (22 June 1999): 53–62; discussion 62–63.

Maslinka, D., and Gajewski, M., "Some aspects of the inflammatory process." *Folia Neuropathologica* 36(4) (1998): 199–204.

Masoro, E. J., Shimokawa, I., and Yu, B. P., "Retardation of the aging process in rats by food restriction." *Annals of the New York Academy of Science* (1990) 1337–352.

Masson, M., "Bromelain in the treatment of blunt injuries to the musculoskeletal system: a case observation study by an orthopedic surgeon in private practice." *Fortschritte der Medezin* 113(9) (1995): 303–06.

McAdam, B. F., et al. "Systemic biosynthesis of prostacyclin by cyclooxygenase (COX)-2: the human pharmacology of a selective inhibitor of COX-2." *Proceedings of the National Academy of Sciences,* 96 (5 January 1999): 272–77.

McAlindon, T. E., et al., "Do antioxidant micronutrients protect against the development of knee osteoarthritis?" *Arthritis and Rheumatism* 39 (1996): 648–56.

McAlindon, T. E., et al., "Relation of dietary intake and serum levels of vitamin D to progression of osteoarthritis of the knee among participants in the Framingham study." *Annals of Internal Medicine* 12(5) (1996): 353–59.

McCarty, M. F., "Enhanced synovial production of hyaluronic acid may explain rapid clinical response to high-dose glucosamine in osteoarthritis." *Medical Hypotheses* 50(6) (June 1998): 507–10.

McColl, K. E. L., et al., "Eradication of helicobacter pylori in functional dyspepsia," *British Journal of Medicine* 319 (1999): 451.

McIlwain, H. H., and Bruce, D. F., *The Super Aspirin Cure for Arthritis.* (New York, NY: Bantam Books, 1999).

McKenna, F., "COX-2: separating myth from reality." *Scandinavian Journal of Rheumatology Supplement* 109 (1999): 19–29.

Mills, W. W., and Farrow, J. T., "The transcendental meditation technique and acute experimental pain." *Psychosomatic Medicine* 43(2) (April 1981): 157–64.

Mindell, E., and Hopkins, V., *Prescription Alternatives* Second Edition. (Los Angeles: Keats Publishing, 1999).

Minor, M. A., "Exercise in the therapy of osteoarthritis." *Rheumatic Disease Clinics of North America* 25(2) (May 1999): viii, 397–415.

"Monograph: Boswellia serrata." *Alternative Medicine Review* 3(4) (August 1998): 306–07.

"Monograph: Bromelain." *Alternative Medicine Review* 3(4) (August 1998): 302–05.

Moreno, B., "Treasures from the sea." *Better Nutrition* (August 1999): 39–41.

Moreno-Reyes, R., et al., "Kashin-Beck osteoarthropathy in rural Tibet in relation to selenium and iodine status." *New England Journal of Medicine* 339(16) (15 October 1998):1112–20.

Mowrey, D. B., and Clayson, D. E., "Motion sickness, ginger, and psychophysics." *Lancet* 20(1) (March 1982): 655–57.

Mukherjee, A., et al., "Predictability of the clinical potency of NSAIDs from the preclinical pharmacodynamics in rats. *Inflammation Research* 45 (1996): 531–40.

Murphy, P. J., Myers, B. L., and Badia, P., "Nonsteroidal anti-inflammatory drugs alter body temperature and suppress melatonin in humans." *Physiology and Behavior* 59(1) (January 1996): 133–39.

Murray, M., and Pizzorno, J., *Encyclopedia of Natural Medicine*. (Rocklin, CA: Prima Publishing, 1991).

Murray, Michael T., *Encyclopedia of Nutritional Supplements*. (Rocklin, CA: Prima Publishing, 1996).

Murrell, G. A., et al., "Nitric oxide: an important articular free radical." *Journal of Bone and Joint Surgery of America* 78 (February 1996): 2, 265–74.

Mustafa, T., and Srivastava, K. C., "Ginger (Zingiber officinale) in migraine headache." *Journal of Ethnopharmacology* 29(3) (July 1990): 267–73.

Nespor, K., "Pain management and yoga." *International Journal of Psychosomatics* 38(1–4) (1991): 76–81.

Nettleton, J. A., "Omega-3 fatty acids: comparison of plant and seafood sources in human nutrition." *Journal of the American Dietary Association* 91 (1991): 331–37.

Newman, N. M., and Ling, R. S. M., "Acetabular bond destruction related to nonsteroidal anti-inflammatory drugs." *Lancet* ii (1985): 11–13.

Nordstrom, D. C., et al., "Alpha-linolenic acid in the treatment of rheumatoid arthritis: a double-blind, placebo-controlled and randomized study: flaxseed vs. safflower seed." *Rheumatology International* 14(6) (1995): 231–34.

Oelzner, P., et al., "Relationship between diseased activity and serum levels of vitamin D metabolites and PTH in rheumatoid arthritis." *Calcified Tissue International* 62(3) (March 1998): 193–98.

Onogi, T., et al., "Capsaicin-like effect of (6)-shogaol on substance P-containing primary afferents of rats: a possible mechanism of its analgesic action." *Neuropharmacology* 3100 (November 1992): 1165–69.

Oparil, S., and Oberman, A., "Nontraditional cardiovascular risk factors." *American Journal of Medical Science,* 317(3) (March 1999): 193–207.

Oxholm, P., et al., "Essential fatty acid status in cell membranes and plasma of patients with primary Sjögren's syndrome: correlations to clinical and immunologic variables using a new model for classification and assessment of disease manifestations." *Prostaglandins, Leukotrienes and Essential Fatty Acids* 59(4) (October 1998): 239–45.

Panush, R. S., "Delayed reactions to foods: food allergy and rheumatic disease." *Annals of Allergy* 56 (1986): 500–03.

Park, K. K., et al., "Inhibitory effects of [6]-gingerol, a major pungent principle of ginger, on phorbol ester-induced inflammation, epidermal ornithine decarboxylase activity and skin tumor promotion in ICR mice." *Cancer Letters* 129(2) (17 July 1998):139–44.

Pelikanova, T., et al., "Insulin secretion and insulin action are related to the serum phospholipid fatty acid pattern in healthy men." *Metabolism: Clinical and Experimental* 38(1989): 188–92.

Pelletier, J. P., "The influence of tissue cross-talking on osteoarthritis progression: role of nonsteroidal anti-inflammatory, drugs." *Osteoarthritis and Cartilage* (4) (July 1999): 374–76.

Perry, G. H., Smith, M. J. D., and Whiteside, C. G., "Spontaneous recovery of the hip joint space in degenerative hip disease." *Annals of Rheumatic Diseases* 31 (1972): 440–48.

Peskar, B. M., et al., "Role of prostaglandins in gastroprotection." *Digestive Disease Science* 43(9 Suppl) (September 1998): 23S-29S.

Petersdorf, R., et al., *Harrison's Principals of Internal Medicine* (New York, NY: McGraw-Hill, 1983).

Pipitone, V. R., "Chondroprotection with chondroitin sulfate." *Drugs Under Experimental and Clinical Research* 17(1) (1991): 3–7.

Pizzorno, J. E., and Murray, M., *A Textbook of Natural Medicine.* (Seattle, WA: John Bastyr College Publications, 1985).

Qiu, G. X., et al., "Efficacy and safety of glucosamine sulfate versus ibuprofen in patients with knee osteoarthritis." *Arzneimittelforschung* 48(5) (May 1998): 469–74.

Rao, C. N., Rao, V. N., and Steinmann, B., "Bioflavonoid-mediated stabilization of collagen in adjuvant-induced arthritis." *Scandinavian Journal of Rheumatology* 12(1) (1983): 39–42.

Rao, C. N., Rao, V. N., and Steinmann, B., "Influence of bioflavonoids on the collagen metabolism in rats with adjuvant-induced arthritis." *Italian Journal of Biochemistry* 30(1) (January/February 1981): 54–62.

Rose, D. P., and Hatala, M. A., "Dietary fatty acids and breast cancer: invasion and metastasis." *Nutrition and Cancer* 21 (1993): 103–11.

Safayhi, H., et al., "Boswellic acids: novel, specific, nonredox inhibitors of 5–lipoxygenase." *Journal of Pharmacology and Experimental Therapies* 261(3) (June 1992): 1143–46.

Sakai, A., et al., "Large-dose ascorbic acid administration suppresses the development of arthritis in adjuvant-infected rats." *Archives of Orthopedic Trauma Surgery* 119(3–4) (1999): 121–26.

Sakamura, F., "Changes in volatile constituents of Zingiber officinale during storage." *Phytochemistry* 26 (1987): 2207–12.

Sander, O., Herborn, G., and Rau, R., "Is H15 (resin extract of Boswellia serrata, 'incense') a useful supplement to established drug therapy of chronic polyarthritis? Results of a double-blind pilot study." *Z Rheumatol* 57(1) (February 1998): 11–16.

Sandoval-Chacon, M., et al., "Anti-inflammatory actions of cat's claw: the role of NF-kappaB." *Alimentary Pharmacology and Therapy* 12(12) (December 1998): 1279–89.

Sangha, O., and Stucki, G., "Vitamin E in therapy of rheumatic diseases." *Zeitchrift fur Rheumatologie* 57(4) (August 1998): 207–14.

Sartor, R. B., "Review article: role of the enteric microflora in the pathogenesis of intestinal inflammation and arthritis." *Alimentary Pharmacology and Therapy* 11 (Suppl 3) (December 1997): 17–22.

Sasaki, S., et al., "Low-selenium diet, bone, and articular cartilage in rats." *Nutrition* 10(6) (November/December 1994): 538–43.

Saso, L., et al., "Inhibition of protein denaturation by fatty acids, bile salts, and other natural substances of a new hypothesis for the mechanism of action of fish oil in rheumatic diseases." *Japanese Journal of Pharmacology* 79(1) (January 1999): 89–99.

Sato, M., et al., "Quercetin, a bioflavonoid, inhibits the induction of interleukin 8 and monocyte chemoattractant protein-1 expression by tumor necrosis factor-alpha in cultured human synovial cells." *Journal of Rheumatology* 24(9) (September 1997): 1680–84.

Schlomo, Y., and Carasso, R.L., "Modulation of learning, pain thresholds, and thermoregulation in the rat by preparations of free purified alpha-linolenic and linoleic acids: determination of the optimal 3 to 6 ratio." *Proceedings of the National Academy of Sciences* 90 (1993): 10, 345–47.

Schmassman, A., "Mechanisms of ulcer healing and effects of nonsteroidal anti-inflammatory drugs." *American Journal of Medicine* 104(3A) (30 March 1998): 43S–51S; discussion 79S–80S.

Schulick, P., *Ginger: Common Spice and Wonder Drug,* Third Edition. (Brattleboro, VT: Herbal Free Press, Ltd., 1996).

Schuna, A. A., "Update on treatment of rheumatoid arthritis." *Journal of the American Pharmaceutical Association* 38(6) (November/December 1998): 728–36.

Sears, B. "Essential fatty acids and dietary endocrinology." *Journal of Advanced Medicine* 6 (1993): 211–24.

Sears, B., and Lawren, B., *Enter The Zone*. (New York: Regan Books, an imprint of HarperCollins Publishers, 1995).

Seeds, E. A., "Role of lipoxygenase metabolites in platelet-activating factor and antigen-induced bronchial hyper-responsiveness and eosinophil infiltration." *European Journal of Pharmacology* 293(4) (7 December 1995): 369–76.

Segal, A. W., et al. "Preliminary evidence for gut involvement in the pathogenesis of rheumatoid arthritis." *British Journal of Rheumatology* 25 (1986): 162–66.

Shanna, S., Prasad, A., and Anand, K. S., "Nonsteroidal anti-inflammatory drugs in the management of pain and inflammation: a basis for drug selection." *American Journal of Therapeutics* 6(1) (1 January 1999): 3–11.

Sharma, S. S., and Gupta, Y. K., "Reversal of cisplatin induced delay in gastric emptying in rats by ginger (Zingiber officinale)." *Journal of Ethnopharmacology* 62(1) (August 1998): 49–55.

Sharpe, R., "Several Deaths Show a Link to Celebrex." *The Wall Street Journal* (20 April 1999).

Shiratori, K., Watanabe, S., and Takeuchi, T., "Effect of licorice extract on release of secretin and exocrine pancreatic secretion in humans." *Pancreas* 1(6) (1986): 483–87.

Silveri, F., et al., "Serum levels of insulin in overweight patients with osteoarthritis of the knee." *Journal of Rheumatology* 21(10) (October 1994): 1899–902.

Simon, L. S., "The evolution of arthritis anti-inflammatory care: where are we today?" *Journal of Rheumatology* 26 Suppl 56 (April 1999): 11–17.

Simon, L. S., et al., "Preliminary study of safety and efficacy of SC-58635, a novel cyclooxygenase-2 inhibitor." *Arthritis and Rheumatism* 41 (1998): 1591–1602.

Simopoulos, A. R., "Omega-3 fatty acids in health and disease and in growth and development." *American Journal of Clinical Nutrition* 54(3) (September 1991): 438–63.

Smith, C. J., et al., "Pharmacological analysis of cyclooxygenase-1 in inflammation." *Proceedings of the National Academy of Sciences* USA 95(22) (27 October 1998): 13, 313–18.

Smith, M. D., Gibson, R. A., and Brooks, P. M., "Abnormal bowel permeability in ankylosing spondylitis and rheumatoid arthritis." *Journal of Rheumatology* 12 (1985): 299–305.

Sobel, D., Klein, A. C., and Bland, J., *Arthritis: What Exercises Work.* (New York, NY: St. Martin's Press, 1995).

Solomon, L., "Drug-induced arthropathy and necrosis of the femoral head." *Journal of Bone and Joint Surgery* 55B (1973): 246–51.

Srivastava, K. C., "Aqueous extracts of onion, garlic and ginger inhibit platelet aggregation and alter arachidonic acid metabolism." *Biomedica Biochimica Acta* 43(8–9) (1984): S335–46.

Srivastava, K. C., "Isolation and effects of some ginger components on platelet aggregation and eicosanoid biosynthesis." *Prostaglandins, Leukotrienes, and Medicine* 2–3 (December 1986): 187–98.

Starbuck, J., "Herbal pain relief: nature to the rescue." *Better Nutrition* (May 1998): 50–56.

Steffen, C., and Menzel, J., "Basic studies on enzyme therapy of immune complex diseases." *Wiener Klinische Wochenschrift* 12:97(8) (April 1985): 376–85

Steffen, C., and Menzel, J., "Enzyme breakdown of immune complexes." *Zeitschrift Rheumatologie* 42(5) (September/October 1983): 249–55.

Steffen, C., et al., "Enzyme therapy in comparison with immune complex determinations in chronic polyarthritis." *Zeitschrift fur Rheumatologic* 44(2) (March/April 1985): 51–56.

Stewart, J. J., et al., "Effects of ginger on motion sickness susceptibility and gastric function." *Pharmacology* 24(2) (1991): 111–20.

Stone, et al., "Inadequate calcium, folic acid, vitamin E, zinc, and selenium intake in rheumatoid arthritis patients: results of a dietary survey." *Arthritis and Rheumatism* 27(3) (December 1997): 180–85.

Surh, Y. J., Lee, E., and Lee, J. M., "Chemoprotective properties of some pungent ingredients present in red pepper and ginger." *Mutation Research* 402(1–2) (18 June 1998): 259–67.

Taussig, S., "The mechanism of the physiological action of bromelain." *Medical Hypotheses,* 6 (1980): 99–104.

Tenenbaum, J., "The epidemiology of nonsteroidal anti-inflammatory drugs." *Canadian Journal of Gastroenterology* 13(2) (March 1999): 119–22.

Tetlow, L. C., et al., "Vitamin D receptors in the rheumatoid lesion: expression by chondrocytes, macrophages, synoviocytes." *Annals of Rheumatic Diseases* 58(2) (February 1999): 118–21.

Tewari, S. N., and Wilson, A. K., "Deglycyrrhizinated licorice in duodenal ulcer." *Practitioner* 210 (1973): 820–25.

Tixier, J. M., et al., "Evidence by in vivo and in vitro studies that binding of pycnogenols to elastin affects its rate of degradation by elastases." *Biochemical Pharmacology* 33(24) (1984): 3933–39.

Truss, C. O., "The role of Candida albicans in human illness." *Journal of Orthomolecular Psychiatry* 10 (1981): 228–38.

Tuncer, S., et al., "Trace element and magnesium levels and superoxide dismutase activity in rheumatoid arthritis." *Biological Trace Element Research* 68(2) (May 1999): 137–42.

Van den Ende, C. H., et al., "Dynamic exercise therapy in rheumatoid arthritis systematic review." *British Journal of Rheumatology* 37(6) (January 1998): 677–87.

Vane, J. R., et al., "Cyclooxygenases 1 and 2." *Annual Review of Pharmacology Toxicology* 38 (1998): 97–120.

Vassilopoulos, D., Camisa, C., and Strauss, R. M., "Selected drug complications and treatment conflicts in the presence of coexistent diseases." *Rheumatic Disease Clinics of North America* 25(3) (August 1999): 745–77.

Vassilopoulos, D., et al., "Gamma-linolenic acid and dihomo-gamma-linolenic, acid suppress the CD-3 mediated signal transduction pathway in human T cells." *Clinical Immunology and Immunopathology* 83(3) (June 1997): 237–44.

Vellini, M., et al., "Possible involvement of eicosanoids in the pharmacological action of bromelain." *Arzneimittelforschung* 36(1) (1986): 110–12.

Verma, S. K., et al., "Effect of ginger on platelet aggregation in man." *Indian Journal of Medical Research* 98 (October 1993): 240–42.

Versteeg, H. H., et al., "Cyclooxygenase-dependent signaling: molecular events and consequences." *FEBS Letter* 445(1) (19 February 1999): 1–5.

Virgili, F., Kobuchi, H., and Packer, L., "Procyanidins extracted from pinus maritima (Pycnogenol): scavengers of free radical species and modulators of nitrogen monoxide metabolism in activated murine RAW 264.7 macrophages." *Free Radical Biology and Medicine* 24(7–8) (May 1998): 1120–29.

Walker, J. A., et al., "Attenuation of contraction-induced skeletal muscle injury by bromelain." *Medicine and Science in Sports and Exercise* 24(1) (January 1992): 20–25.

Weatherby, C., and Gordin, L., *The Arthritis Bible*. (Rochester, VT: Healing Arts Press, 1999).

Westacott, C. I., et al., "Synovial fluid concentration of five different cytokines in rheumatic diseases." *Annals of Rheumatic Diseases* (September 1990) 676–81.

Whitehouse, M. W., et al., "Anti-inflammatory activity of a lipid fraction (Lyprinol) from the NZ green-lipped mussel." *Inflammopharmacology* 5 (1997): 237–46.

Wilder, R. L., "Adrenal and gonadal steroid hormone deficiency in the pathogenesis of rheumatoid arthritis." *Journal of Rheumatology Supplement* 44 (March 1996): 10–12.

Williams, C. A., "The flavonoids of Tanacetum parthenium and T. vulgare and their anti-inflammatory properties." *Phytochemistry* 51(3) (June 1999): 417–23.

Williams, P. J., Jones, R. H., and Rademacher, T. W., "Reduction in the incidence and severity of collagen-induced arthritis in DBA/1 mice, using exogenous dehydroepiandrosterone." *Arthritis and Rheumatism* 40(5) (May 1997): 907–11.

Willis, A. L., *Handbook of Eicosanoids, Prostaglandins and Related Lipids*. (Boca Raton, FL: CRC Press, 1987).

Wilson, D. E., "The role of prostaglandins in gastric mucosal protection." *Trans Am Clin Climatol Assoc* 107 (1995): 99–113.

Wolfe, S. M., and Sasich, L., "Before the FDA's arthritis drugs advisory committee on the nonsteroidal anti-inflammatory drug (NSAID) Celecoxib (Celebrex)." Statement given on behalf of the Public Citizen's Health Research Group (1 December 1998).

Woolf, C. J., et al., "Cytokines, nerve growth factor and inflammatory hyperalgesia: the contribution of tumor necrosis factor alpha." *British Journal of Pharmacology* 1 (12 June 1997): 3, 417–24.

Wu H., et al., "Effect of dry ginger and roasted ginger on experimental gastric ulcers in rats." *Chung Kuo Chung Yao Tsa Chih* 15(5) (May 1990): 278–80, 317–18.

Yamahara, J., et al., "Cholagogic effect of ginger and its active constituents." *Journal of Ethnopharmacology* 13(2) (May 1985): 217–25.

Yamahara, J., et al., "Gastrointestinal motility enhancing effect of ginger and its active constituents." *Chemical and Pharmaceutical Bulletin,* (1990).

Yamahara, J., et al., "Inhibition of cytotoxic drug-induced vomiting in suncus by a ginger constituent." *Journal of Ethnopharmacology* 27(3) (December 1989): 353–55.

Yamahara, J., et al., "The anti-ulcer effect in rats of ginger constituents." *Journal of Ethnopharmacology* 23(2–3) (July/August 1988): 299–304.

Yashiro, N., "Clinico-psychological and pathophysiological studies on fasting therapy." *Sapporo Medical Journal* 55(2) (1986): 125–36.

Yoshikawa, M., et al., "Stomachic principles in ginger. III. An anti-ulcer principle, 6–gingesulfonic acid, and three monoacyldigalactosylglycerols, gingerglycolipids A, B, and C, from Zingiberis rhizoma originating in Taiwan." *Chemical Pharmacy Bulletin* (Tokyo) 42(6) (June 1994): 1226–30.

Zaphiropoulos, G. C., "Rheumatoid arthritis and the gut." *British Journal of Rheumatology,* (1986): 138–40.

Zurier, R. B., et al., "Gamma-linolenic acid treatment of rheumatoid arthritis." *Arthritis and Rheumatism* 39(11) (1996): 1808–17.

Index

Aspirin, 17, 24–25, 27, 101
Asthma, 13, 27
Auranofin, 34
  side effects, 35
Autoimmune arthritis. *See*
  Rheumatoid arthritis.
Autoimmune disorders, 8–10, 27, 43
Autonomic nervous system, 106
Ayurvedic medicine, 45, 79, 81, 91, 96
Azathioprine, side effects, 35

Back exercises, 124–125, 128
Back-leg extension, 123
Back-of-wrist stretch, 121
Back pose, 128
Back press, 128
Bacterial infection, 11, 13, 36
Balance muscles, training, 128–129
Ball squeese, 126
Beta-carotene, 69, 71–72
Betaine HCL, 50
Bicycling, 117
Bifidus bacteria, 63
Bile, 48, 89
Bioflavonoids, 39, 69
Birth control pills, 63
Bliddal, Henning, 87
Blood, 17–18
Blood circulation, 111
Blood clotting, 48, 89–90
Blood glucose. *See* Blood sugar.
Blood sugar, 20, 52
Blood vessels, 17–18
Boat scoot, 123
Bone, 75
  density, 33
Boswellin, 96
Bow and arrow, 127
Bowel movements, 50
Bread, 53
Breathing, 114
  deep, 115
Bromelain, 70, 74–75
Bursae, 4, 6
Bursitis, 6, 11
Buttocks exercises, 127

Caffeine, 26

Calcium, 75
Cancer, 17, 89–90, 107
Candida albicans, 62–63. *See also* Yeast.
Capillaries, 47
Capsaicin, 100–101
Carbohydrates, 20
Carbonic-anhydrase inhibitors, 27
Cardiovascular fitness, 113–118
  warm-up routines for, 119–120
Carotenes, 71–72
Carotenoids, 71–72
Carpal tunnel syndrome, 6, 11
Cartilage, 4–5, 8, 75, 93–96, 114
Cat stretch, 125
Cat's claw, 96
Celecoxib, 25, 28, 29
Cetyl myristoleate (CMO), 100
Chemicals
  in cleaning supplies, 55
  in foods, 54
Chest exercises, 122, 126–127
Chi, 104
Chinese medicine. *See* TCM.
Cholesterol, 48
Chrondroblasts, 4
Chondrocytes, 85
Chondroitin sulfate, 95–96
Chromium, 53
Chronic fatigue syndrome (CFS), 6
Chyme, 47
Clonidine, 91
Clostridium, 49
Cobra, The, 124
Coffee. *See* Caffeine.
Colitis, ulcerative, 13
Collagen, 4, 68, 70, 76
Collagenases, 70
Colon. *See* Intestine, large.
Complementary medicine, 11, 67
  finding a practitioner, 131–132
  vs Western medicine, 39–41
Confucius, 81
Connective tissues, 3–4, 8–9. *See also*
  Bursae; Cartilage; Fasciae; Fat;
  Ligaments; Tendons.
Constipation relief, 50
Conventional medicine. *See* Western
  medicine.

About the Author

Earl Mindell, R.Ph., Ph.D., is an internationally recognized expert on nutrition, drugs, vitamins, and herbal remedies. He is the author of more than fifty books, including the *New Vitamin Bible, Prescription Alternatives, Soy Miracle, New Herb Bible, Anti-Aging Bible, Peak Performance Bible,* and *The Diet Bible.* He is a registered pharmacist, master herbalist, and a professor of nutrition at Pacific Western University in Los Angeles. He conducts nutritional seminars around the world and lives in Beverly Hills, California.